BEAUTY WISDOM

BEAUTY WISDOM

Bharti Vyas

with
Claire Haggard

Thorsons
An Imprint of HarperCollins*Publishers*

Thorsons
An Imprint of HarperCollins*Publishers*
77–85 Fulham Palace Road
Hammersmith, London W6 8JB

Published by Thorsons 1997

1 3 5 7 9 10 8 6 4 2

© Bharti Vyas 1997

Bharti Vyas and Claire Haggard assert the moral right to
be identified as the authors of this work

A catalogue record for this book
is available from the British Library

ISBN 0 7225 3399 3 (HB)
ISBN 0 7225 3663–1 (PB)

Printed and bound in Italy by
New Interlitho Italia, SpA

I dedicate this book to my beloved husband, Raja, who has always given me the freedom to follow my path in life. He, along with my daughters, Shailu and Priti, have given me uncon-ditional love, support, encouragement and belief. Without them I would be nowhere. I also dedicate this book to my late dear mother, Pushpaben, and to my aunt, Vijyaben, who has been a second mother to me. They were both an inspiration to me for, as Indian women, they were both far ahead in their era. They taught me the value of succeeding in what you want to do without jeopardizing family stability and happiness. And to my grandchildren, who have always inspired me to carry on.

And, to my co-author, Claire Haggard, goes my most sincere thanks. *Beauty Wisdom* would not have happened without her. She, of all people, understood my philosophy.

CONTENTS

ACKNOWLEDGEMENTS

ALL my thanks go to: my sons-in-law, Bharath and Parag, who are both a tower of strength; my brother Satish, who has helped and supported me with all the ventures I have undertaken; my dear friend, Jane Goldsmith, who was initially a client but on whom I now rely for her tremendous advice and encouragement; the late Margot Walton Clarke, who was my PR consultant until 1992 and who communicated my philosophies so beautifully, which contributed to my success; Janis Raven who continued where Margot left off; Robin Maclear, who introduced me to the Marco Polo cruise lines which opened many doors for me; all the journalists who believe in my therapies and philosophies and who have been very supportive of my work over the years including Jenny Baden, Eve Cameron, Elizabeth Rees-Jones, Chrissie Painell, Lisa Podmore, Joan Thornycroft, Vicki Wisdom and Newby Hands, M. Cidesco, a lady whom I respect greatly and who, when I told her of my intention to write a book, gave me a great deal of encouragement and support which inspired me to progress; Jane Fisher who was so generous with her time and support; Ray Cochrane College and Balgit Suri, who trained me and gave me a firm basis of knowledge on which I could build my therapies and who provide me with continuous support; David Harris, MB, MRCP, for his encouragement and belief in my therapy and its benefits in the medical world; Ben Woodhouse, the talented young artist, for his support; Eileen Campbell, the Managing Director of Thorsons and Wanda Whiteley, who both believed in my abilities and have guided me through the past year, giving me continuous support and encouragement all the way; Lord and Lady Beaverbrook, who have encouraged and advised me throughout; Len Bernie who, 18 years ago, inspired me to reach for higher things, told me that I had a great deal of potential and made me believe in myself and my abilities; Caroline Shott, my marketing consultant, who has guided and supported me and kept my feet firmly on the ground with her sound, focused advice; and finally, all my staff who have become like part of my family and have rallied around me each day helping me with research and advising me, including Magda Reggio, Anouk Auchere, Tessa Fitch, Vaishally Patel, Angela Almeida, Lucy Lebow and Najma Abbars.

Beauty on the *outside*

INTRODUCTION

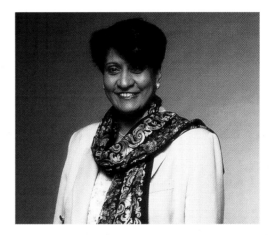

I N THE 15 years that I have been running my own beauty clinic in London, I have set out to teach my clients how to carry on their beauty care at home. By writing *Beauty Wisdom*, I hope to bring home this practical philosophy to everyone.

There is a fundamental truth about beauty care: *beauty on the outside begins on the inside*. The information in the second part of this book is not intended to be a biology lesson. It is there to help you to make the connection between your inner health and outer beauty, between inner vitality and outer radiance.

The routines which I describe in this book are easy to learn and will soon seem as natural as brushing your teeth.

The main bulk of the book consists of a Top to Toe guide. Starting with the scalp, I have taken each part of the body in turn, listing the most common problems I encounter and offering practical assistance and, where relevant, a suitable skincare and make-up routine. I am only too aware of the limitations imposed by family commitments and a hectic lifestyle and have, therefore, tried to put forward suggestions which are simple, practical, affordable and –

above all – effective. I hope you enjoy *Beauty Wisdom* and that it will help you to take better care of yourself and your family. And remember, if you *know* you are looking good, you can take on the world!

Bharti Vyas

begins on the inside

THE ESSENTIALS

Hands are sensitive *and*

MOST beauty clinics put pressure on their clients to commit to a course of treatments because they know that they cannot effect any lasting change in a single session. My philosophy has always been to allow people to come and go as they please, but to give them the practical know-how to continue and consolidate the therapy they receive at my clinic in their own homes.

If people agree to keep up the routines I give them, I know that they will see improvements, not just in their appearance, but in their general health and wellbeing. If they go on to make these routines a way of life, they will develop a new-found confidence in their looks and discover stores of untapped energy. Helping people to make the most of themselves is one of the great satisfactions of my work.

A word of warning: do not expect instant results. The purpose of the Home Therapy treatments is to activate and rebalance some of the body's key internal systems – most importantly the circulation – in areas where they are proving ineffective. The efficient functioning of this internal machinery is what determines whether you look and feel your best. Some problems respond quickly to attention, while others will need many weeks of consistent repetition. Make these routines a regular habit so that they become preventative *as well as* curative.

In order to do the following routines – and yourself – justice, you need to set aside an hour a week for an initial period of six weeks. At first it might seem unrealistic, even self-indulgent. Once you start noticing a difference, however, not just in your complexion and the texture of your skin, but in the way that you feel, you will be bending over backwards to make the time. An hour a week is a *minimum* commitment.

MOVE INTO MASSAGE

Massage used to be the preserve of the rich and is still regarded as something of a luxury. Traditionally, wealthy people would employ masseurs to assist in the task of preserving their youthful appearance by giving their system a 'cleansing' work-out.

Our hands are highly sensitive and powerful beauty tools, with the ability to influence the workings of our internal body and, therefore, the health of our skin. When applying certain massage techniques using different parts of our hands, we ensure

powerful beauty tools

that our skin is nourished properly by regulating the blood supply to the cells *and* guard against stagnation and toxic build-up by assisting the process of lymphatic drainage (*see* page 164) – both essential steps in the quest for firm, clear, young-looking skin. Activating important acupressure points which lie just beneath the skin's surface (*see* page 28) provides us with many additional benefits.

We have all felt the soothing effect of massage on tired and tense muscles, and the relief that comes when muscles are relaxed and blood is able to flow through them freely once more. Regular massage is equally important for our joints, helping to relieve congestion and disperse waste which could, over time, cause deterioration and reduced mobility. The physical act of self-massage also has a toning effect on fingers, forearms and biceps.

It is a great knack to be able to relax and soothe yourself at the end of a long, hard day or punishing week. These routines will help every bit of your body to unwind fully, at the same time as restoring internal balance. Don't begrudge the time it takes – enjoy it, revel in it – it is entirely for your benefit.

SIMPLE TECHNIQUES

In order to manipulate any area of the body effectively, we need to learn how to use our hands. These are the three main techniques we will be applying.

Finger Ball

The balls of our fingers are very richly supplied with nerve endings and, therefore, capable of detecting any change in the skin's texture, as well as in the muscles and tissue beneath. These 'sensors' allow us to read our skin more accurately and handle it with greater sensitivity.

The balls of the fingers are used to stimulate nerve endings and galvanize the body's transport systems – blood and lymph – into action using small circular movements in a specified area. The rule is to apply pressure to a depth that feels comfortable. If the area you are working on is tender, you will need to start with a light touch, then apply more pressure as the discomfort begins to ease. The balls of the index finger and thumb are used to stimulate acupressure points (*see* pages 28–35).

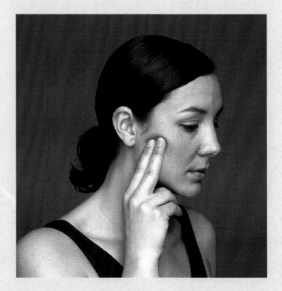

Palming

The palms of our hands contain many nerve junctions which radiate a lot of heat. They have a powerful and healing magnetic action which can be used to correct imbalances in other parts of the body.

The superficial stroking action, using only the palms of your hands, is particularly useful on swollen joints and those areas of the body which cannot take vigorous stimulation. When repeated over several minutes, palming triggers off the parasympathetic nervous system (that is – not under the voluntary control of the brain), whose job it is to redress the balance within the body and restore all functions to normal after a crisis. In other words, this gentle palming action can work deeper than the deepest massage.

Pinching

Small pinches use the thumb and index finger to work a small area such as the forehead. Large pinches require all four fingers plus the thumb and are useful for substantial muscles such as the trapezius on the back of the shoulder or the large muscle groups on the thighs. Contrary to how it may feel, pressure eases nerves. So persevere with tender spots. Remember – the thumb exerts more pressure than the fingers.

Pinching is a fast action, designed to irritate and, therefore, activate the nerve endings in the skin. The brain responds to the mild pain sensation by increasing circulatory activity, which revives the cells and helps to siphon off the waste via the lymph (*see* page 165).

Note: do not massage the site of an open wound or areas where the skin is sore or infected.

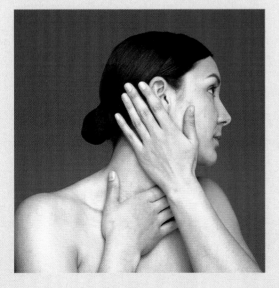

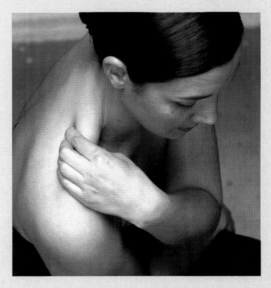

OIL

Oil is used in these routines to encourage a smooth, rhythmic action and to avoid dragging the skin. Apply just enough to allow your fingers to glide smoothly over your skin. Soak a cotton wool ball with oil and then wipe it over the area you are going to work on. You may end up using a little more if your skin is very dry.

BEFORE YOU BEGIN

There are no hard and fast rules concerning the best time to carry out your Home Therapy. Since you will need to set aside a good hour, weekday mornings may well be difficult. Weekend mornings or evenings will probably be best. Ideally, start or finish with a good soak in the bath, so add that in to your time calculations.

Before beginning, bring a comfortable, up-right chair into your chosen room and make sure that you have a free surface for oils, cotton wool, a towel and maybe a comb. Line up a bath mat to rest your feet on once they have been oiled. Fill a glass with water to sip away at. The room should be warm, as you will be uncovering different parts of your body as you work.

There is no need to place yourself in front of a mirror, in fact it is probably more distracting. The aim is to get your fingertips to connect with the nerve endings beneath the skin. If you are unable to see what you are doing and whether you are doing it correctly, you are more likely to rely on your hands and your sense of touch will become more acute.

Sit well back in the chair with your bottom tucked under, tummy pulled in and shoulders relaxed and back (*see* page 120). Do not slump in the middle, as this will prevent you from breathing well and so reduce the amount of oxygen available to your cells.

Check your position at the beginning of each routine and correct it if necessary. You will need to adjust your position slightly to carry out some procedures and to stand up to do others. Assume the sitting position unless stated otherwise.

Breathe slowly and deeply throughout and stop to take a few deep breaths in between routines. This will also help to keep your muscles relaxed.

Almond oil is highly nutritious, versatile and pretty easy to get hold of.

Olive oil is useful for excessively dry skin and lubricating larger expanses.

Jojoba is a wonderful massage oil, especially for the face, although it is fairly costly. Very easily absorbed, it seems to suit highly sensitive skins as well as oily complexions. It also has a longer shelf life than most other oils. Mix a little jojoba in with a more workaday oil, such as sunflower or grapeseed, for massage purposes.

As far as quality is concerned, cold-pressed is best.

HEAD & SHOULDERS

Set aside 30 minutes for the full facial therapy. This is the minimum time required to awaken the nerve endings and get the draining process underway – some of the mechanisms responsible for imparting a youthful glow and firm tone to the skin.

Think of the time it takes as an investment and a saving. If you visit a beauty clinic regularly, you could reduce your visits and maintain the effects in between times by doing your own treatment at home. If you don't, you will be receiving a lot of the benefits you would from a professional facial without any financial outlay. The difference with this facial is that, by tuning into key acupressure points located on the face, you will be promoting the health of other parts of the body at the same time as 'servicing' your face.

Before beginning, make sure that your hair is well back off your face and that you have removed any jewellery or clothing which might get in the way. Remove your bra or pull the straps down. Pour a few tablespoons of your massage oil into a bowl and apply a light film all over your face, shoulders and neck.

FRONT SHOULDERS

All facial treatments start at the collarbones. By stimulating an acupressure point on the stomach meridian (energy channel) and linking into the lung meridian, this routine will calm tension in the stomach and increase the oxygenation of the body.

Position the first two fingers of each hand on your collarbones, at the point where they meet your breastbone. Press the balls of your fingers firmly into the flesh immediately beneath your collarbones and release (*see* below).

Continue this movement as you progress out towards the shoulder joint. This should take about four moves. Return in the same manner to the breastbone. Repeat five times.

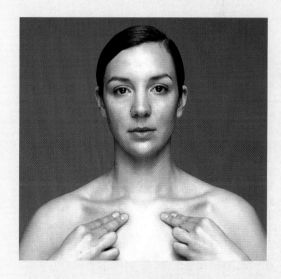

BACK SHOULDERS

The trapezius muscle, a thick triangular-shaped muscle which lies behind your shoulder (*see* page 118), is one of the most common sites for tension to build up. Using the three middle fingers of one hand, massage thoroughly the part of the muscle located behind the opposite shoulder with small circular movements. Repeat on the other side. The greater the store of tension, the deeper you will need to work to release it. Increase pressure gradually though – contracted muscles need to be coaxed gently out of their rigid state.

Now place your thumb in the hollow behind your collarbones and, using all four fingers, 'pinch' all over the muscle repeatedly (*see* below). This is meant to exert real pressure on the nerve endings and may be quite uncomfortable if the muscles are in spasm – that is, permanently contracted. Carry on for as long as you can, then repeat the movement on the other side. The same vigorous pinching action, with your thumbs pointing downwards, can be used on the back of the neck moving up towards the hairline.

Continue for at least five minutes, switching between strokes and shoulders. Do not reduce the time spent on this routine – unless this area is relaxed, any therapy you carry out on your face will be wasted.

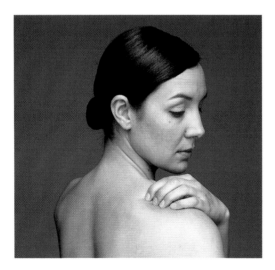

NECK

We have to be very gentle in our treatment of our neck due to the delicate nature of the tissue, the underlying thyroid gland and the proximity of the voice box. This routine uses the magnetic field of the palms to influence the metabolism via the thyroid and adjoining parathyroid glands, as well as keeping the skin firm and supple.

Massage your neck from left to right in a rhythmical, upward-stroking motion, with one hand following the other. If you start with the palms at the base of the neck, you should finish with the forefingers up under the chin (*see* Palming, page 7). Continue for two or three minutes. Next, pinch gently all over the front and sides of your neck for a further minute. Use your right hand for the left side and vice versa. Finish with an additional two minutes of stroking. Since we cannot work at any depth on the neck, we have to work for longer.

JAWLINE

Position your thumbs just beneath your chin and the balls of your fingers on top (*see* above right). Now pinch your way along the lower jawbone until you reach the earlobes, applying greater pressure at the corner of the jawbone and just beneath the earlobes (*see* above right centre). You should work deeply enough to feel the jawbone. Aim to cover the distance in four pinches and repeat the sequence ten times.

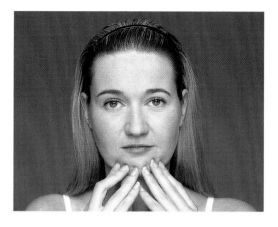

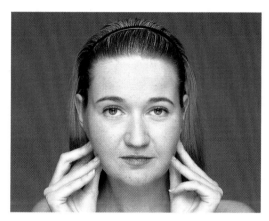

CHEEKS

Using the first two fingers of each hand, work along the underside of the cheekbones, pressing the balls of your fingers gently against the bone and then releasing them (*see* Finger Ball, page 6). Work out towards the point where your cheekbones and upper jawbones meet, then come back towards the centre, four or five moves in each direction. Repeat ten times.

You may find tender spots, signalling little pockets of stagnation. These should

disappear and your face acquire more definition after a few weeks, as the increased circulation disperses trapped toxins and fatty deposits. If you are carrying extra weight on your face, regular stimulation will stop it from looking heavy and bring back a glow to your cheeks.

SINUS POINTS

This exercise will help to clear or prevent blocked sinuses. When you are 'bunged up', this affects the eyes as well as the skin surrounding the nose, which becomes puffy and lifeless. Once you clear the sinus points, you will automatically feel and look better as well as regaining your sense of smell.

Using the balls of your index fingers, apply pressure to the muscles on either side of the nose, starting at the bridge and moving down to the nostrils (*see* below). Your fingers should be pointing inwards so that you feel cartilage rather than bone. Continue for about one minute.

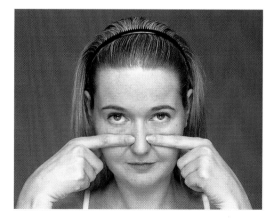

EYES

The skin around the eyes is the thinnest anywhere on the body and one of the first places on our face to show signs of ageing. In addition to keeping it moisturized, the following routine will help to avoid stagnation in the tissue by stimulating the lymphatic circulation to drain any fluids and toxins which may have accumulated.

Close your eyes and feel the bony rims of your eye sockets. Starting at the outer edge, use your third fingers to trace around the rims of the sockets, applying more pressure across your brow and at the point where the eyebrow meets the side of the nose (*see* sequence right). Do at least ten 'laps' at a steady pace, working on both eyes simultaneously. Only use your third fingers, as this will prevent you from exerting too much pressure on the delicate eye tissue.

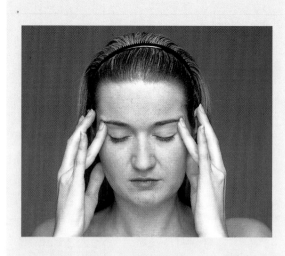

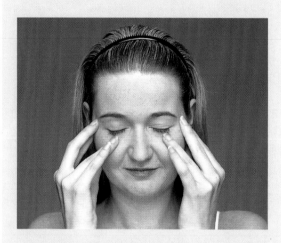

FOREHEAD

Position your thumbs just above the outer edge of your eyebrows and your index fingers above the inner edge. Pinch in a rhythmical fashion up towards the hairline and back again. Now place your thumbs on your temples and repeat. Continue for a couple of minutes. Although this is a very shallow pinch – almost a flick, as there is so little flesh to get hold of – it is effective in encouraging regeneration and preventing lines.

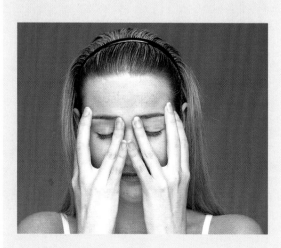

SCALP

A thorough scalp massage will help to release tension from the scalp – a major factor in undernourished, out-of-condition hair, as it interferes with the all-important blood supply to the hair follicles. It will also promote a feeling of general wellbeing (*see* pages 45–46 for full instructions).

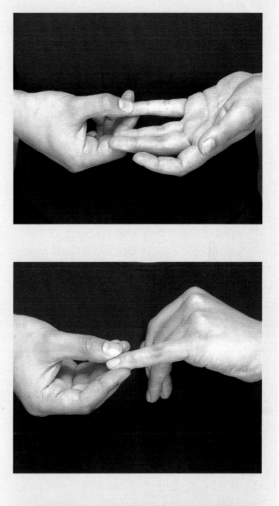

UPPER EXTREMITIES

Remove any jewellery and apply almond oil all over your fingers, hands and arms. Do your left hand first if you are right-handed, and vice versa. Allow seven or eight minutes to complete these exercises.

HANDS

Our hands become surprisingly congested. This routine will help to clear the blockages and relieve any aches and soreness.

With your thumb on top and your index finger in a supporting role, massage the balls of your fingers, your nails and your finger joints (*see* right). Push your thumb along the furrows between the tendons that run down the back of your hand and glide it up towards the wrist to 'drain' the hand (*see* page 102). You will need to work from the outside for the first three movements and from the thumb side for the last one. Pinch the web between each finger before you start each gliding action.

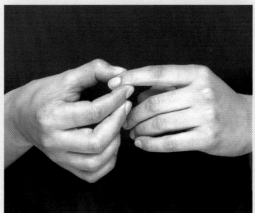

While your thumb is manipulating the top of your hand, your fingers should be draining your palm in an upwards motion. If they seem congested, apply extra pressure to the muscle pads on the outside of the hand.

WRISTS

Wrap the fingers of the working hand around the outside of the hand you are treating and massage all over the top side of your wrist joint with your thumb, using small circular movements. Really roll your thumb around the bones on either side. Now turn your wrist over and cradle it in the other hand while you do the underside.

FOREARMS

The muscles of the forearms can become sore and strained as a result of carrying children or lugging heavy bags, for example. This routine will help to ease any discomfort and keep the forearms slender by guarding against fluid retention. Bend your arm and wrap your fingers around its underside, just above the wrist (*see* above right). Divide your arm into outer and inner 'tramlines' and use your thumb, pressing and gliding for short bursts and then releasing, to drain the tissue to the elbow in two sections (*see* bottom right). Your palm should not come into contact with your arm.

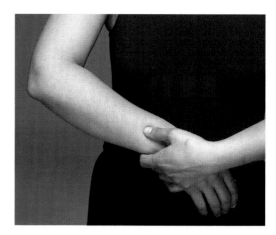

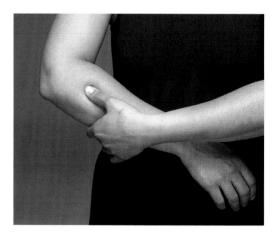

ELBOWS

Rest your hand on your abdomen and use the thumb and finger balls of the working hand to massage your elbow joint, making sure that you get into all the grooves. Apply sustained pressure to the acupressure point located at the outer edge of the elbow crease when the elbow is held at a right angle (*see* page 29). This will act as a wonderful tonic to your entire system.

UPPER ARMS

Using all four fingers and your thumb, start on the outside of your upper arm at the elbow and work your way up to the shoulder, pinching your flesh as you go. Next tackle the inside of the arm, with your thumb on the inside and your fingers reaching around your arm. Now repeat the movement. If your muscles are slack and underused, this may feel quite tender. Continue until the area seems well-stimulated.

SHOULDERS

Feel the rim of the shoulder joint and, with your thumb on the front and the balls of your fingers on the back, manipulate it gently.

Rub in any excess oil using the palms of your hands, then repeat the steps on the other arm.

LOWER EXTREMITIES

Lubricate the skin of your feet and legs with oil, being careful not to over-oil the feet, as they will become slippery and difficult to work on.

In the sitting position, cross one leg over the other so that you are sitting with one ankle resting on the other thigh. This enables you to reach your feet easily,

although you may be a bit stiff to begin with. Always start with your 'weaker' side first (your right foot if you are left-handed and vice versa) and work with the opposite hand unless otherwise specified.

FEET

Any attention you pay to your feet will be handsomely rewarded, as the benefits will extend throughout the body via the reflexology zones (*see* page 129).

Massage thoroughly all over your toes and your toenails using your thumb and index finger. Pinch the web between your toes and, with the sole facing downwards, drain your feet in the same way as you did your hands, using your thumb on the upper side and your three middle fingers on the sole (*see* below). Now give the soles of your feet a good rub.

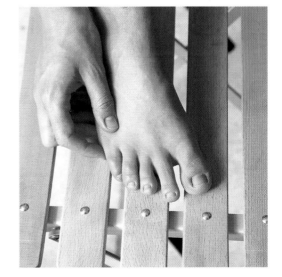

ANKLES

Adjust your position so that the outside of your foot is propped higher up your thigh, sole uppermost. Use the balls of your fingers to apply pressure to the different parts of your ankle, thumb on the inside and fingers on the outside. Work the area thoroughly, not forgetting the spot above the Achilles tendon.

CALVES

The muscles of the calves are seldom relaxed since they are rarely off duty. To relieve tension, slide your ankle a little way back down your thigh and massage the outside of the muscles using the forefingers, while your thumb does

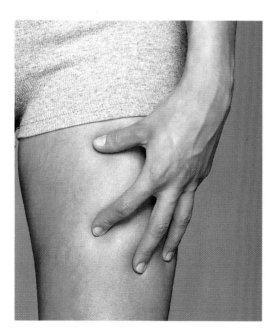

the inside. The stroke is a deep pinching action. Reverse the position of your fingers and thumbs and repeat the movement. Next, with thumb and forefinger on either side of the shin bone, glide and drain up towards the knee. Note: if you suffer from varicose veins, ignore the above instructions and palm the lower leg instead, using gentle sweeping strokes from ankle to knee.

KNEES

Stand up and grasp lightly behind one knee with the fingers of both hands. Position your thumbs on top and manipulate the joint both front and back until it is thoroughly warmed. Use your fingertips gently to ease the area around the kneecap.

THIGHS

Still in a standing position (possibly with one foot resting on the edge of a chair), massage all over your raised thigh by rotating your fingers and thumbs and applying a firm pressure. There are several large muscles in the upper legs, so you need to be systematic to make sure that you don't miss a section. Reduce the pressure over thread veins and go easier if you have fine skin.

Now repeat these routines on the other leg.

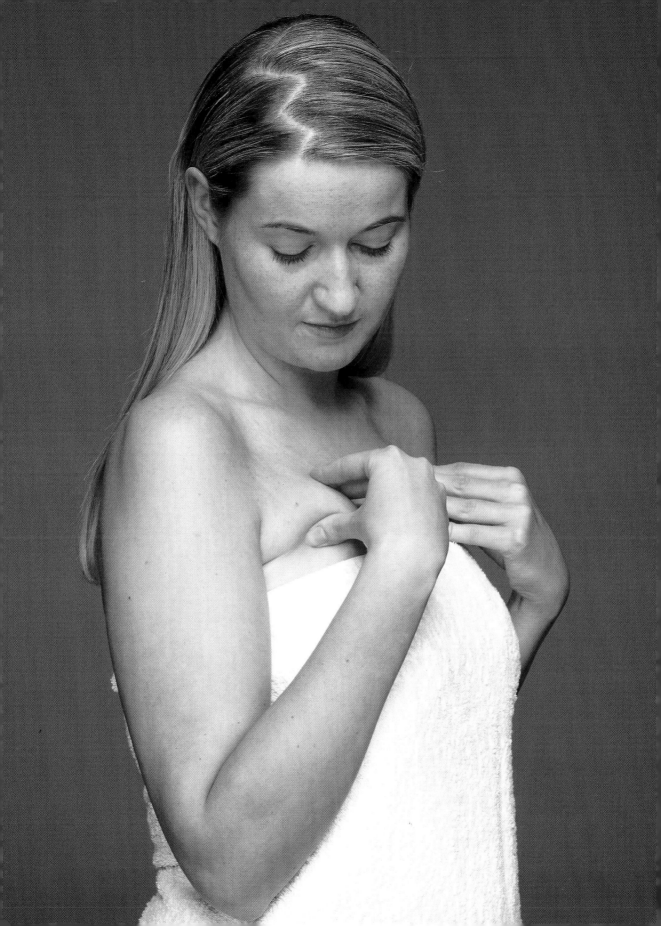

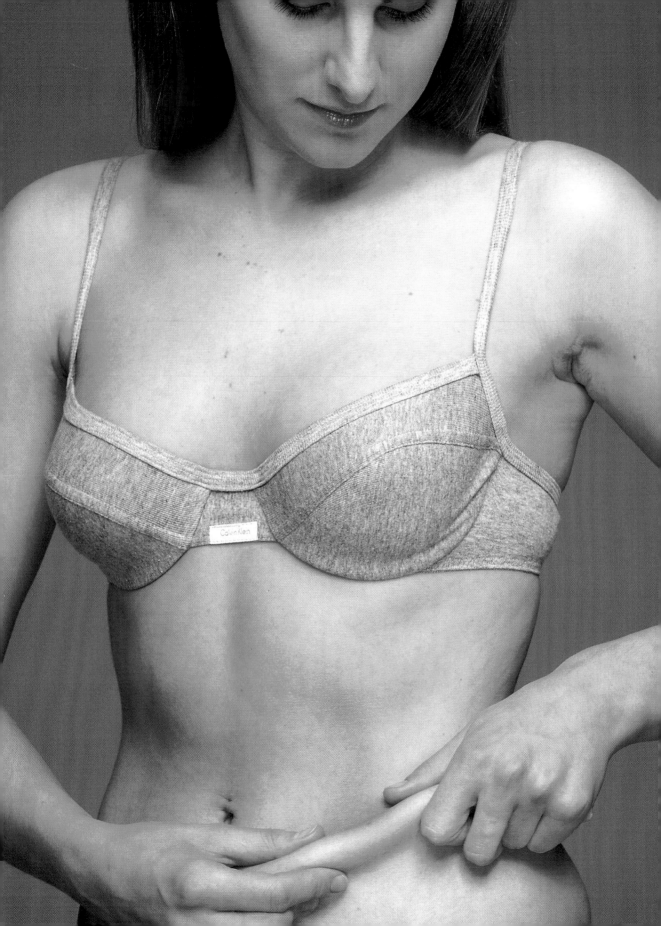

THE TRUNK

Warm the oil between your palms and apply a light covering all over your trunk. Stand with your feet shoulder-width apart, your bottom tucked under and your tummy pulled in. Your shoulders should be relaxed and back. Allow eight to ten minutes to complete these routines.

BUST

There is no muscular tissue within the breasts themselves to keep them firm, but the neighbouring muscles help to provide support. This exercise will help to condition the underlying pectoral muscles and the diaphragm (*see* illustration on page 173), which is prone to accumulate fatty tissue. It will also encourage deeper breathing.

Anchor your thumbs just inside your armpits and stimulate the area above the breasts (at the point where the bra and bra straps would meet) using deep pinches (*see* page 17). Continue for a minute or so. Now put one hand on top of one breast and use the other hand to massage underneath with large, deep, circular movements. Repeat 20 times on each side.

STOMACH

Check that you are in the correct standing position and that you have not allowed your abdominal muscles to collapse forwards – the contraction helps to drain the tissue. Using firm pressure and a slow circular motion, massage your abdomen with the palms of your hands for a couple of minutes, avoiding the area around the navel. Now grasp the flesh in big pinches and drain to the side (*see* left).

HIPS AND BUTTOCKS

Breathing slowly and deeply, tighten your buttock muscles and pinch firmly all over your hips and bottom, using your thumb and all four fingers. Hold for a count of 10, then release. Repeat 30 times. This is an intensive therapy which will be particularly valuable if you tend to put on weight on your bottom. Initially your finger muscles may not quite be up to the task, but persevere. You will only receive the full benefits when your fingers are strong enough to pinch deep into the muscles.

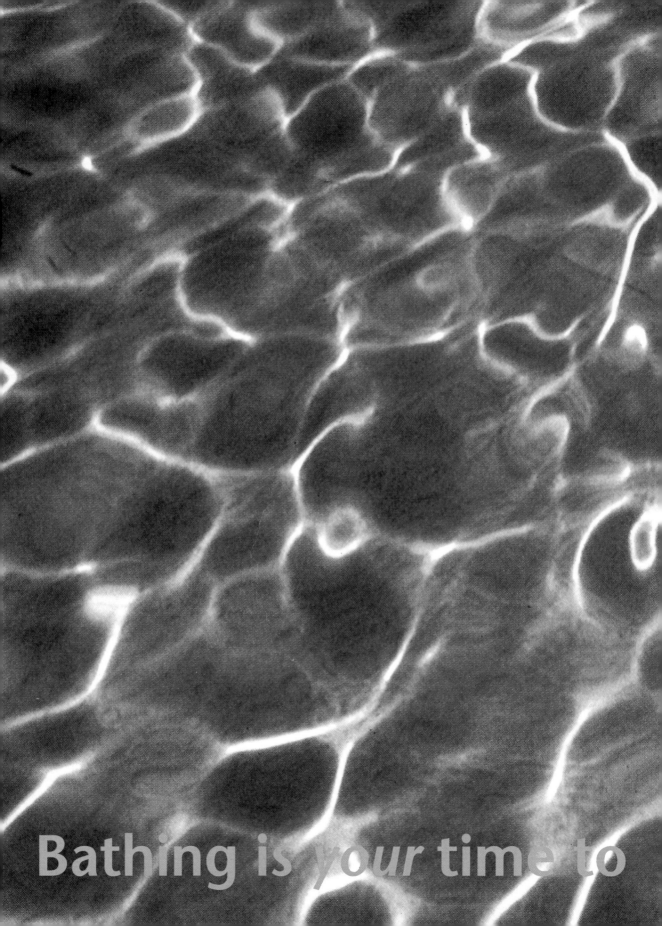
Bathing is *your* time to

I OFTEN hear women saying that they don't have time to relax because they're too busy. It is exactly such women who most need the benefits proper relaxation can bring.

Many of us require superhuman stamina to do all that is demanded of us – to bring up a family and keep the various elements of a household ticking over, often at the same time as holding down a demanding job. Our health and well-being are therefore a top priority – hence the importance of making time to look after ourselves. If we don't make a point of it, no one else will.

mind, our nerves, our posture and our sleep, as well as our body's ability to carry out its many vital functions effectively.

The best action we can take is preventative. Whether performing the juggling act described earlier or grappling with totally different pressures, it is essential that you have a complete break from time to time, to give your mind and body the opportunity to unwind and recharge.

LIE BACK AND RELAX!

Relaxing is one of the most effective ways of counteracting stress. It diffuses the accumulated physical and psychological pressure so that, when you go back into battle, you feel refreshed and your load feels lighter. This in turn will make you far more able to withstand any stress you do experience, since it will help you to experience it in a more positive way. Stress should also then not invade your life in quite the same way. And stress can be very invasive, affecting our state of

One of the most therapeutic treatments we can give ourselves is a long, relaxing soak in the bath. Children are also exposed to different kinds of stress and, if you teach them how to dispel such tension, you will be equipping them with a valuable means of self-protection and survival for later in life. Beneficial bathing habits will also help keep their skin clear and encourage them to wind down in preparation for a good night's sleep. Play your children some soothing music or read them a story during their bath time, so that they come to associate it with relaxation. Teenagers,

relax and relieve stress

despite their bathroom-hogging reputations, should be given their chance to wallow too.

I have put together a Home Spa treatment designed for every member of the family. If you follow my routine regularly, I believe it will make a big and positive difference to your life.

Children can be treated to the full routine once in a while, although you may want to reduce the quantity of salts to one or two handfuls and replace the body scrub with a face cloth for the exfoliating massage.

BATHTIME WITH BHARTI

Try to give yourself at least 30 minutes in the bath, once or twice a week. If you suffer from specific skin problems, such as psoriasis or eczema, or have sleeping difficulties, make it a daily routine. Stress, diet, injury and illness can all have a traumatizing effect on body tissues, which, initially, makes them less able to absorb and make use of the minerals contained in the salts. It is therefore important to take more frequent baths to begin with, until you notice some improvement.

I believe passionately in the health benefits of Dead Sea salts. The very high concentration of minerals in the salts, tiny quantities of which enter the body through the pores, have a natural therapeutic action on the skin and benefit the body as a whole. Their effect on the external body is to boost the skin's excretory function by dissolving the dehydrated dead cells which accumulate on the surface. This speeds up the elimination of the body's waste and has a smoothing and refining effect on the skin.

Of the 28 naturally occurring minerals in the salts, three are particularly valuable for our internal health: potassium, which regulates the fluid balance within our bodies and the circulation of blood and lymph; magnesium, our body's main 'nerve food'; and bromide, which has a calming and restorative effect on the system. Because these substances are part of the body's own make-up, they are immediately 'recognized', absorbed and put to use.

Regular salt baths can correct all sorts of imbalances within the body. They encourage gentle detoxification of the system and reduce fluid retention in the tissues, which can assist weight loss and relieve problems affecting the joints. They act as an antidote to the potentially damaging effects of stress and strengthen our resistance to disease. They also safeguard that cornerstone of our health and well-being: sleep. By quelling anxiety and restoring calm, a salt bath taken at the end of a gruelling day both aids and enhances sleep.

GET READY

First, prepare everything you are going to need – your cassette player if you want to listen to some soothing music or, perhaps, the book you are reading, plus a towel to pat your hands dry. An untidy or cluttered bathroom can be a distraction in itself, so straighten things up in advance.

Make sure that you have a flannel available and a large towel or some newspaper to cover the floor. The room needs to be comfortably warm. If you like the idea, light three or four candles around the bathroom to evoke a little atmosphere. The gentle, flickering light is more restful to the eyes than an electric bulb and helps the body begin to unwind.

SIMPLE STEPS

Start with the Scalp

Begin by oiling your scalp (*see* pages 45–46 for full details of scalp massage). When you have completed the scalp massage, wrap your hair in a towel or a shower cap. Massage your scalp regularly at least once a week, when you are due to wash your hair.

Exfoliation

Now move on to the exfoliating treatment, designed to boost your circulation, loosen any dead skin cells and moisturize your skin in preparation for the mineral therapy which is to follow. Even if you

take salt baths more frequently, this part of the routine should only be carried out once a week, although your skin will always benefit from a light covering of almond oil before you begin your soak.

Stand on the floor covering or in the empty bath and rub the All-purpose Oatmeal Scrub (*see* page 36) into your skin, first over your trunk, then onto arms, legs, neck, face and even behind your ears. This is very invigorating in itself and you will notice your skin becoming warm and pink in response. Pay special attention to hard skin on elbows, knees, soles and heels, on which the scrub has a remarkable softening effect. Massage the paste into finger and toenails, working right into the cuticles. Shower the paste off before you run your bath.

If you find this too messy, substitute a mild commercial exfoliant. In between the weekly body-exfoliating sessions, concentrate your efforts on rough or callused patches of skin. The natural exfoliating properties of the salts are usually sufficient for male bathers, who tend to be more efficient in sloughing off dead skin cells than their female counterparts.

The Magic of Minerals

Now fill up the bath and add three or four handfuls of Dead Sea salts plus a squirt of mineral shower gel for your mineral therapy. If you suffer from a dry skin condition such as eczema, start with as little as a teaspoon of salts, increasing gradually as tolerance builds up.

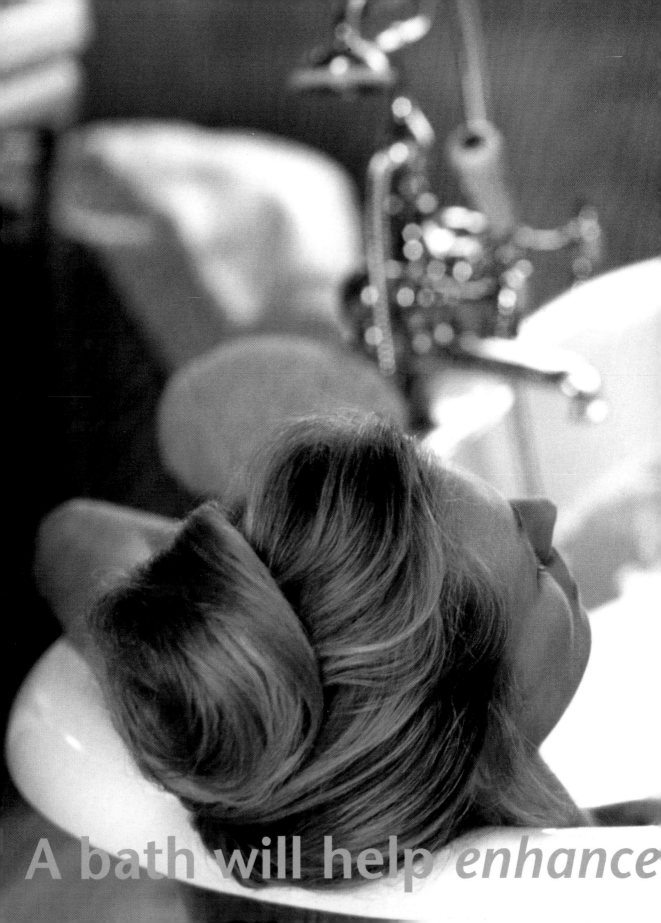
A bath will help *enhance*

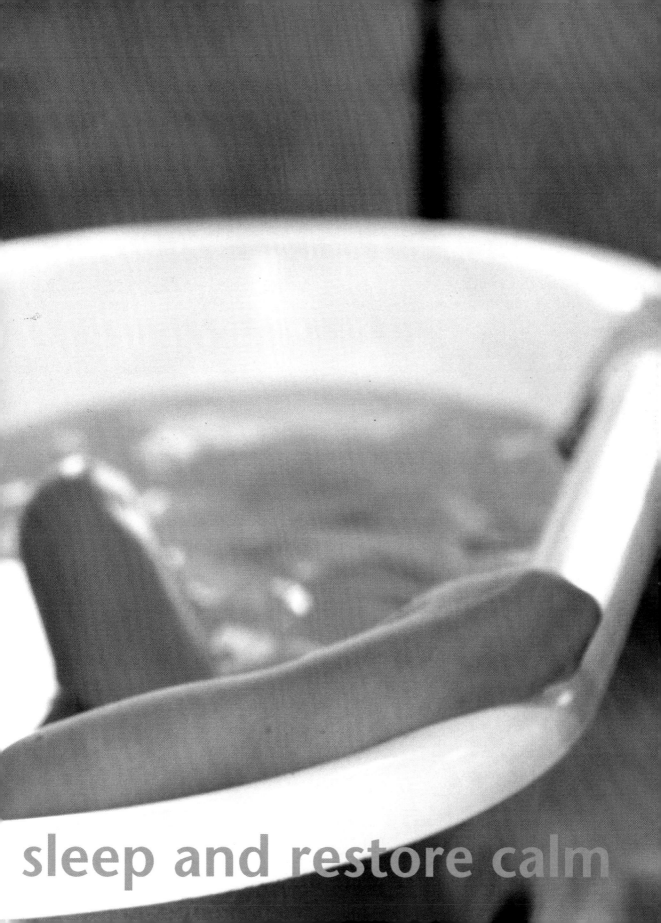

sleep and restore calm

The water should be pleasantly warm, so that you feel inclined to linger. If the bath is too hot, it will stimulate rather than relax your system and can also have a dehydrating and slackening effect on the skin, as well as damaging fragile capillaries.

Try adding five drops of essential oil to the water. **Lavender** is a wonderfully soothing aroma which helps ease aches and pains as well as soothing the nervous system. It also works on the mucous membranes of the nose to give an instant feeling of relaxation. Alternatively, try **sandalwood**. This aphrodisiac is useful for dispelling nervous tension, lifting depression and relieving insomnia. It is extremely well-suited to dry skins.

Submerge yourself in the bath and soak for a good 10 minutes. Your face and scalp will also benefit from being immersed briefly at some point, so remove your cap or towel and take a quick dip. Next, gently rub your face cloth all over your body, especially on areas of hard skin. Use the cloth to push back the cuticles around your finger and toenails and relax for a further 10 minutes. Remember to shower the salts off before you get out of the bath. Finish by applying a good mineral body lotion to further hydrate your skin.

FINISHING UP

Now go straight to bed or relax under a warm cover. Long hair can be tied back in a loose plait. Use an old towel to protect your pillow from the coconut oil. When you wash your hair – after a brief interlude, or when you wake in the morning – lather it twice to remove all visible traces of the oil. I recommend using a mineral shampoo, which should be left to work on the scalp for 10 minutes before rinsing. If you have your bath before going to bed, the therapy can go on working overnight, assisting the repair process that is underway when the body is at rest.

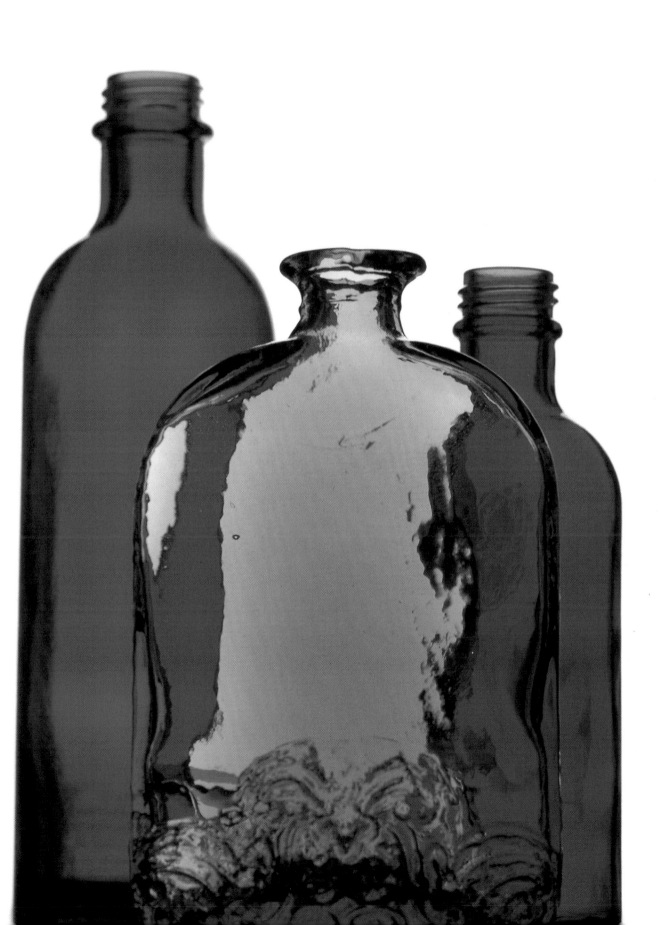

ACUPRESSURE is another way of using our hands to enhance our health and vitality. According to Chinese Medicine, the energy or vital force inhabiting every individual flows along established channels or meridians. These are connected to the organs and systems of the body. When this flow of energy is interrupted, it creates an imbalance within the body which is manifested on the outside as a problem or symptom. By stimulating the pressure points of the meridians which lie just beneath the surface of the skin (acupressure points or acupoints), the natural harmony can be restored.

I have found acupressure to be a very valuable beauty tool. I began to incorporate it into massage routines because I knew that, by applying pressure to certain, congested spots on the skin, I could achieve much greater results than with a generalized massage. The benefits to the skin were deeper and longer-lasting.

The effect of regular acupressure on key points is to fine-tune our internal machinery, increase our energy levels and resistance to illness, while enhancing, directly or indirectly, different aspects of our appearance. It is easy to see the connection between a sluggish digestive system or inefficient circulation and the health of the skin, or how a constant level of pain or stiffness could distort your posture as well as your facial expression. You can help to relieve such problems by administering your own acupressure treatment.

CONTRAINDICATIONS

Acupressure is a very safe form of treatment entirely free of side effects. Even if you end up stimulating the wrong point, it will not do you any harm. However, it is important to follow certain guidelines.

■ Do not apply pressure to skin which is bruised, broken or inflamed, to open wounds or to varicose veins.

■ Avoid acupressure treatment when under the influence of drink or recreational drugs.

■ The following points should not be stimulated in pregnancy: Large Intestine 4, Spleen 6, Urinary Bladder 60.

How to restore your

APPLYING PRESSURE

Precise instructions and illustrations are given to help you locate the points. With practice, you will be able to home in on the spot instantly although, initially, you may feel rather at sea and wonder what it is you are feeling for. A mild pain sensation will often confirm that you are in the right place.

Prolonged pressure on the acupoints is not advisable, as the nerves carrying therapeutic impulses can become over-accustomed to the stimulus. Instead, each acupoint should be treated by applying a deep pressure, then releasing it. Sometimes it is more effective to position the thumb or fingertip at an angle to the point and then apply pressure. Carry out this 'pumping action' 60 times – for the duration of approximately one minute.

The homoeostatic points (*see* below) should be activated twice daily, morning and evening, to maximimize their preventative as well as their curative potential. If you can get into the habit of doing it first thing in the morning and last thing at night, it will become an automatic part of your daily routine. Treatment using the other points can be administered as the need arises.

HOMOEOSTATIC POINTS

These five points are designed to assist the process of homoeostasis in our bodies. This is necessary to maintain a stable environment and to regulate the body's most important functions – blood pressure, body temperature and blood sugar levels. These are prone to be disturbed by a variety of mental and physical factors, including stress, anxiety and lack of sleep. Regular stimulation of these points will bolster your immune system, reduce allergic sensitivity and keep you going through the most difficult times. Don't wait until you're run down – make it a way of life.

LARGE INTESTINE 11 (LI 11)

Location: at the outer end of the skin crease, when the elbow is bent. Support the elbow in the fingers and palm of the opposite hand and apply deep pressure with the thumb.

Benefits: gently cleanses the digestive system and prevents/relieves constipation. Enhances the body's ability to assimilate nutrients from food, kick-starts the metabolism and improves body shape. Tones the skin and enhances the complexion. Improves the mobility of arms and elbows. In conjunction with other points, encourages optimum functioning of all bodily systems.

STOMACH 36 (St 36)

Location: with the knee bent at a right angle, measure four finger widths down

body's *natural* harmony

from the lowest point of the knee. The point is at this level, one finger width towards the outside of the leg. Apply pressure with your index or middle finger.

Benefits: improves circulation through-out the body and acts as a tonic for the digestive system. By aiding digestion, it increases vitality and stamina and enhances general skin tone. Soothes tired, aching legs and feet and relieves knee joint pain.

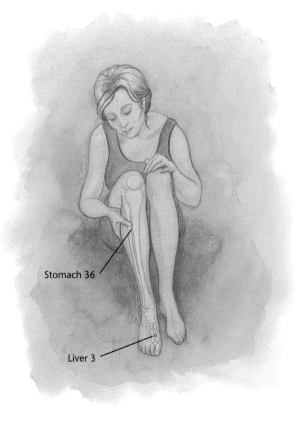

Location of Stomach 36 and Liver 3.

SPLEEN 6 (Sp 6)

Location: four finger widths above the tip of the prominent bone on the inside of the ankle, just behind the shin bone (*see* page 34). Measure with one hand and apply pressure with the middle or index finger of the other. This is where the spleen, liver and kidney meridians meet and is a very powerful acupressure point. Note: avoid during pregnancy.

Benefits: boosts circulation and encourages elimination of excess fluids in the lower body. Raises general energy levels and enhances sexual vitality. Improves digestion and relieves abdominal bloating. Having a balancing effect on hormonal activity, it is useful for treating menstrual problems and pre-menstrual tension (PMT). Increases mobility and relieves pain in legs and feet.

LIVER 3 (Liv 3)

Location: on the upper surface of the foot, approximately two thumb widths below the web between the big toe and the second toe. Place your fingers under your feet and use your thumb to apply pressure in the hollow between the bones.

Benefits: improves liver function and boosts the immune system. Relieves effects of stress and toxins in the body and regulates blood pressure. Reduces irritability sometimes referred to as 'liverishness' and combats depression. Improves circulation in legs, relieves cramp and aching muscles and helps prevent varicose veins.

GOVERNING VESSEL 14 (GV 14)

Location: when the head is bent forwards, two vertebrae stand out prominently where the top of the spine meets the base of the neck. The point is located in-between the two vertebrae. Reach over your shoulder with one hand and apply firm pressure with the tip of your first or second finger, with your neck in an upright position.

Benefits: highly effective in preventing illness, this point will also reinforce the other homoeostatic points.

SEDATIVE POINTS

These are the points that soothe the nerves and calm the mind. They are of immense value in times of stress or on any occasion when you feel anxious or agitated, as they can help to minimize the internal and external symptoms by stimulating the discharge of tranquil-lizing hormones.

GOVERNING VESSEL 20 (GV 20)

Location: in the middle of the top of the head, halfway between the ears. Position thumbs on the tips of the ears, to get your bearings, then apply pressure using your middle finger.

Benefits: this is the most powerful sedative point in the body. Balances emotions and sharpens mental faculties, as well as improving memory and powers of concen-tration. Very effective in regulating blood pressure and raising general energy levels.

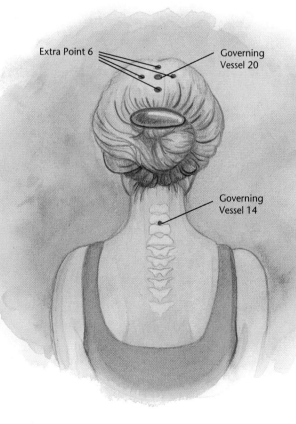

Location of Governning Vessel 14, Governing Vessel 20 and Extra Point 6.

HEART 7 (Ht 7)

Location: draw an imaginary straight line on the palm, starting at the web of the 'ring' (that is, third) and little finger and finishing at the wrist. It lies at the junction of this line and the wrist crease. Support the wrist with the fingers of the opposite hand, with the palm facing upwards, then locate the point with the thumb. Use your thumb to apply pressure with a pumping action for approximately 60 seconds.

Benefits: calms the nervous system and relieves mental tension, anxiety and sleeplessness. A very valuable point if you are trying to give up smoking, as it strengthens the lungs and stimulates the brain to produce a chemical which makes nicotine distasteful.

PERICARDIUM 6 (P 6)

Location: two thumbs widths above the wrist joint, in the centre of the forearm between the tendons. Support the wrist with the fingers of the opposite hand, with the palm facing upwards, then locate the point with the thumb. Use your thumb to apply pressure with a pumping action for approximately 60 seconds.

Benefits: calms the mind and sedates the upper digestive tract. Useful for treating nausea, vomiting (including morning sickness) and heartburn. Eases breathing difficulties triggered by anxiety and helps to relieve insomnia.

LARGE INTESTINE 4 (LI 4)

Location: at the peak of the small mound of muscle created by pressing the thumb and first finger together. Apply firm pressure with your thumb while your fingers support your hand from beneath. Note: avoid during pregnancy.

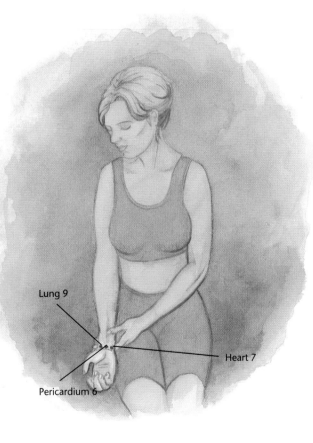

Lung 9

Heart 7

Pericardium 6

Location of Heart 7, Lung 9, Pericardium 6 and 7.

Benefits: sometimes referred to as the 'aspirin point', this general analgesic point is very effective in treating problems affecting the front of the head, the face (including all the sense organs) and the neck. Regulates the function of the lower intestine and promotes elimination. Calms the mind, relaxes the upper body and relieves tension in the neck, shoulders, arms, hands and fingers. Enhances mental function.

GENERAL POINTS

LUNG 9 (Lu 9)

Location: in the shallow depression on the wrist crease at the base of the thumb on palm side. Apply pressure with your thumbs, using a pumping action for approximately 60 seconds.

Benefits: boosts respiratory system and oxygen levels. Strengthens the blood vessels in the body and brings back colour to dull complexions. Improves the suppleness of the wrists and the condition of hands and nails.

SMALL INTESTINE 6 (SI 6)

Location: draw an imaginary line on the back of your hand, starting from the web between your middle and ring finger. The point is found at the junction of the line and wrist. Apply pressure with your thumb using a pumping action for approximately 60 seconds.

Benefits: relieves pain and stiffness in the neck, which helps to improve the posture. Improves the suppleness of the wrists and the condition of hands and nails.

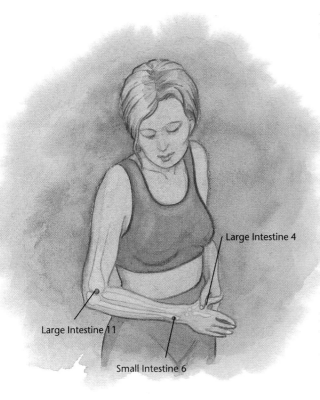

Location of Large Intestine 11, Large Intestine 4 and Small Intestine 6.

PERICARDIUM 7 (P 7)

Location: at the centre of the inner wrist crease, between the tendons. Apply pressure with your thumb using a pumping action for approximately 60 seconds.

Benefits: promotes efficient circulation which improves overall skin tone. Increases vitality and energy. Improves the suppleness of the wrists and the condition of hands and nails.

URINARY BLADDER 60 (UB 60)

Location: in the hollow between the ankle bone and the Achilles tendon, on the outer side of the foot. Wrap the index finger around the ankle and apply pressure with thumb. Note: avoid during pregnancy.

Benefits: improves function of urinary system and boosts immune system. Increases mobility and relieves aches, pains and swelling in the legs, ankles, heels and feet.

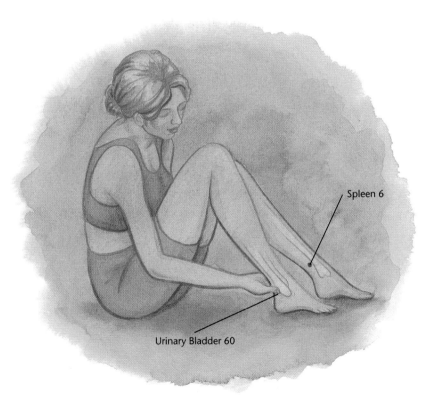

Location of Spleen 6 and Urinary Bladder 60.

GALL BLADDER 20 (GB 20)

Location: at the back of the neck, just above the hairline, in the depression between the bottom of the skull and the neck muscles. Rest your fingers on the back of your head and apply pressure with your thumbs.

Benefits: relieves stiffness and discomfort in the neck and shoulder area.

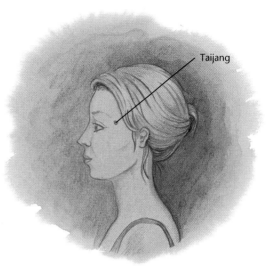

Location of Taiyang.

TAIYANG

Location: one thumb width beyond the eyebrow, in a dip in the skin halfway between the outer edge of the eyebrow and the corner of the eye. Apply circular pressure using your index finger for about a minute.

Benefits: relaxes tense facial muscles and revitalizes expression and complexion.

EXTRA POINT 6

Location: two finger widths above, below and to the left and right of Governing Vessel 20 (*see* page 31). Apply pressure with the first and second finger of each hand using a pumping action for approximately 60 seconds.

Benefits: relieves anxiety and insomnia and balances the mind and emotions.

KITCHEN CUPBOARD TREATMENTS

Here is a collection of instant recipes for traditional cosmetic preparations using basic cooking ingredients. These simple recipes have proved their effectiveness over centuries of use. Apply masks to cleansed skin and remove immediately if you feel any discomfort. Rinse off with warm water and pat skin dry. Moisturize well afterwards. The quantities given are enough for one thick application.

Gentle Facial Exfoliator (Sensitive Skin)

2 heaped tsp fine oatmeal
2 tsp double cream

Combine ingredients, apply to skin and rub with a very light action using the balls of your fingers, then rinse off. Do not apply sustained pressure to any particular spot.

Cleansing Mask (Congested Skin)

2 heaped tsp gram flour
1 tsp water
1 tsp honey

Thick, sticky consistency. Apply to affected areas and leave for five to seven minutes.

All-purpose Oatmeal Scrub

2 tbs finely ground oatmeal
1 tbs almond oil

Directions as above. Also suitable for all-over body use.

Stabilizing Face Mask (Sensitive Skin, Acne Rosacea, Premature Wrinkles)

1 heaped tsp gram flour
1 tsp double cream
2 tsp water and a pinch of salt

Gram or chickpea flour, a cosmetic staple in Indian households, is prized for its ability to nourish and cleanse the skin. Buy it at health shops, large supermarkets and Asian stores. This mask is of a thick and creamy consistency. Apply to skin and leave for 10 minutes before rinsing off.

Healing Mask

2 tsp honey
1/4 tsp fine sea salt
1 tsp turmeric

Thick paste. Apply to spots every evening and leave on for up to 30 minutes or even overnight. Once the spots have cleared, this treatment can be used preventatively as a face pack once a month.

Exfoliator (Irregular Pigmentation)

2 heaped tsp fine oatmeal
2 tsp honey
$1/4$ tsp lemon juice

Sloppy consistency. Leave on for 10 minutes.

Eye Mask

2 tsp juice grated cucumber
1 tsp powdered milk

Thick paste. Close eyes and cover upper and lower eyelids. Leave for 10 minutes then wipe off with moist cotton wool.

Firming Mask (Podgy Droopy Cheeks)

2 heaped tsp gram flour
2 tsp water
$1/2$ teaspoon honey

Creamy paste. Leave on for 15 minutes.

Lemon-based Mask (Excess Hair)

1 tsp lemon juice
1 tsp honey

Very liquid. Smooth the paste on in the direction of hair growth and leave for 10 minutes.

Eczema Mask

2 tsp gram flour
2 tsp almond oil
$1/4$ tsp salt

Smooth and fairly liquid consistency. Apply to affected area and leave for 10 minutes.

Nourishing Cheek Mask (Combination Skin)

2 tsp gram flour
2 tsp honey

Gooey consistency. Spread the paste over your cheeks and leave for 10 minutes.

Nose Mask

$1/2$ tsp gram flour
$1/2$ tsp honey
a pinch of salt
a few drops of lemon juice

Cover your nose with the paste, allowing it to overlap onto your cheeks. Leave for 5–10 minutes.

■ As soon as you feel the tell-tale tingling sensation of a cold sore, hold an ice compress against the area. Once the sore has erupted, dab on **lemon juice** mixed with a pinch of **salt**. Dilute with water if it seems too concentrated.

■ In addition to dislodging dead skin cells, **honey** is valued for its soothing, healing, emollient and mildly antiseptic properties. Use the runny variety. Avoid the masks containing honey if you are allergic to pollen and grasses.

■ Particularly well suited to dry, irritated and sensitive skins, **oats** and **oatflakes** have a gentle but deep cleansing action and can correct skin imbalances. If you cannot get hold of ground oatmeal, porridge oatflakes crumbled between your fingers will do.

■ **Double cream** has a composition not unlike a rich moisturizer and is naturally well endowed with vitamin A, as well as useful amounts of vitamins D and E – a natural skin food.

■ **Lemon juice** is a great cleanser and healer with anti-bacterial properties. A useful natural bleaching agent, it also helps to restore the skin's acid balance.

■ **Salt** is a powerful cleanser and neutralizer of bacteria, as well as a natural exfoliator.

■ The healing power of **turmeric** is renowned in India, where it is sprinkled onto cuts to speed up the clotting and repair process. Combined with other ingredients in a mask, it is very effective in clearing the complexion.

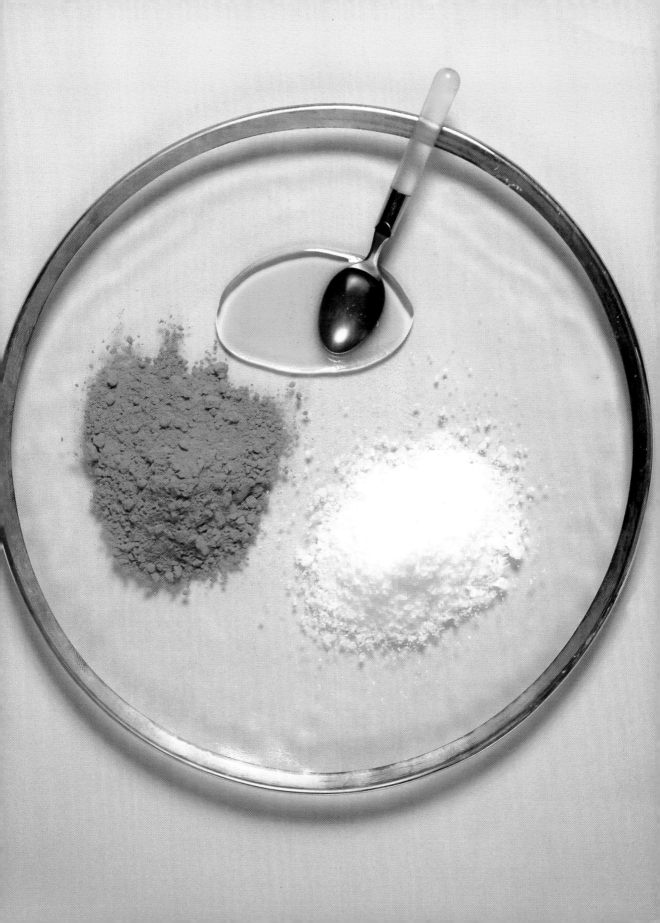

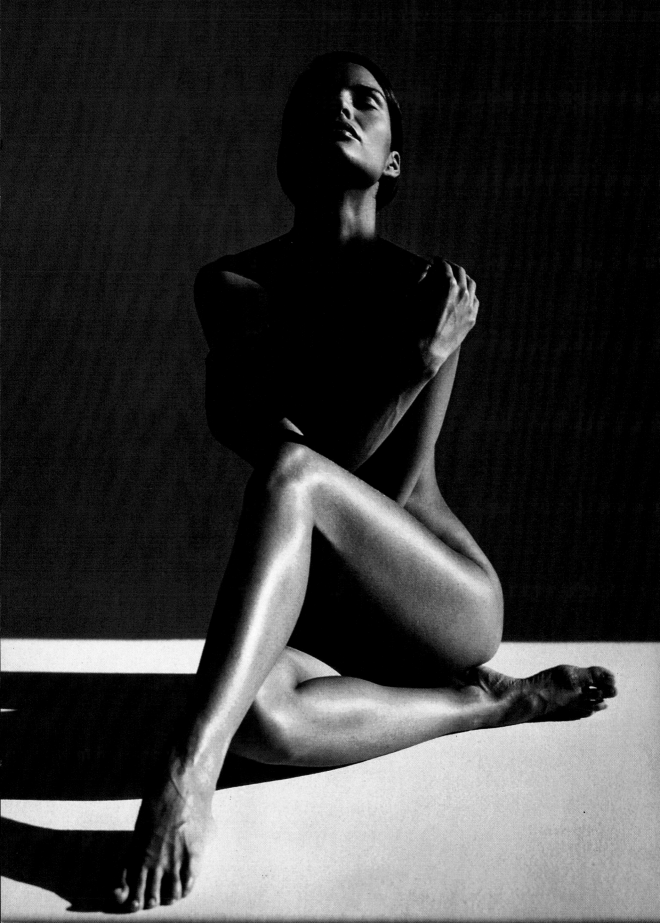

TOP TO TOE

OUR hair has the power to lift or depress our spirits. Beautiful hair is as much a source of pride for a man as it is for a woman and we spend millions of pounds teasing and taming our crowning glory in an attempt to make the most of what we've got. Yet the real secret lies in understanding how to nurture our hair and improve its condition from the *inside*.

A healthy scalp should be firm and supple and move easily when you try to manipulate it. If you've forgotten how malleable a problem-free scalp can be, lay your hands on the head of a willing child to remind yourself. If you are still in any doubt about the state of your scalp, look at your hair. Is it lustrous? Does it 'bounce'? If not, the chances are that your scalp is in need of attention.

As a therapist, I make a strong connection between the condition of someone's hair and the condition of their scalp. Each strand of hair emerges from a follicle imbedded in the scalp, which is fed and watered by the blood and lymph circulating through the tissue. Our hair grows automatically unless our body is exposed to a huge shock or trauma. The condition of our hair, however, depends on the quality of the nutrients and the general state of health within our bodies. Stress, tension in the scalp, neck and shoulder area, hormonal imbalances, heredity, eating and dieting habits all have a direct impact on the growth and condition of our hair.

SCALP

Poor circulation to the scalp is at the root of many hair problems. In order to have a healthy head of hair, the tens of thousands of follicles crammed into this thick covering of skin need to be properly nourished. Good blood flow and brisk lymphatic circulation to and from your scalp 'feed' hair and prevent toxic build-up.

Make your hair your

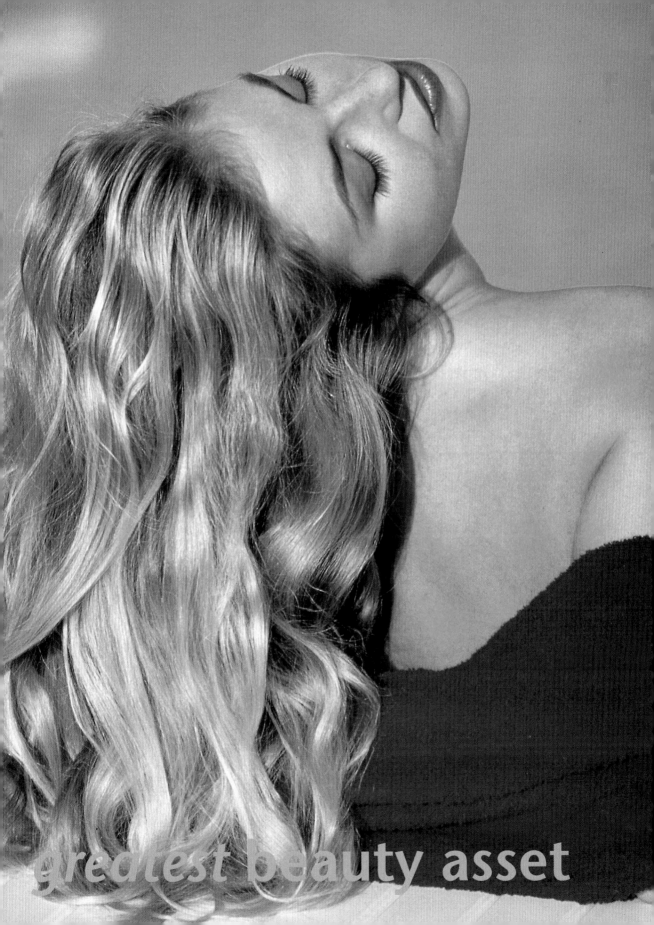

greatest beauty asset

COMMON PROBLEMS

The most common problems I encounter include scalps which are:

- Oily – due to overactivity of oil-producing sebaceous glands in the scalp, influenced by hormones and heredity.

- Dry – resulting from the underactivity of sebaceous glands in the scalp, linked to poor circulation generally but occasionally due to a deficiency of zinc or essential fatty acids in the body.

- Scaly – due to a build-up of dead cells on the scalp caused by stress, dandruff, psoriasis or eczema.

- Itchy – caused by the accumulation of dead skin cells due to poor circulation.

- Pimply/spotty – a symptom of congestion due to poor circulation resulting in bacteria breeding on the scalp.

- Tight (as though the skin is stuck to the scalp) – often a symptom of tension, although hormonal activity and a sedentary lifestyle may cause the circulation of blood and lymph to become sluggish and stagnation to occur.

- Spongy – long-term stagnation results in toxic build-up and retention of fluid beneath the scalp. Makes the head feel heavy and can cause headaches around the temples and on top of the head.

- Smelly – a result of bacteria breeding on the scalp which can give off a pungent smell. PH imbalance due to internal causes is at the root of this problem.

WHAT TO DO

The most effective way to keep your scalp in good working order is to massage it regularly with oil. A head massage may be a luxury in the Western world, but in Asian culture, where great store is set by the condition and thickness of a person's hair, it is part and parcel of the barber's trade. In Indian households it is quite traditional for families to earmark one day a week for communal scalp massages.

> A scalp massage is a wonderful therapy for mind and body, capable of clearing your head, lifting your spirits and evaporating stores of tension, at the same time as looking after one of your greatest beauty assets – your hair.

The physical impact of regular massage on your scalp is to keep the maximum number of follicles active and increase the strength and diameter of each hair. The movements of your hands and fingers act on the blood vessels beneath the surface (increasing the blood supply to the area) and on the follicles themselves. Manipulating your scalp also helps to release tension, which improves the general flow of blood and rectifies any underlying imbalances. As an extra bonus, during a massage the natural scalp oils are spread evenly along the length of the hair instead of remaining at the roots.

Coconut oil is ideal for hair massage. What is more, the invisible coating left after washing acts as a protective shield, locking moisture into the hair shaft as well as providing a barrier against the sun, heated styling appliances and hair processing chemicals. Available from most chemists and Asian food stores, it is solid at room temperature. To liquefy it, stand the container in a bowl of boiling water for 10–15 minutes or microwave for about one minute before beginning the massage. Alternatively, if you only have time for a quick massage, scoop a fingerful out of the pot and rub between your hands to melt. Olive and almond oil are both possible substitutes.

The Bharti Vyas Scalp Massage

Before you start, measure out 3 tablespoons of the liquefied oil into a bowl. Halve the quantity if your hair is oily or very fine.

- Begin by activating the following group of acupressure points on the crown of your head: Governing Vessel 20 and Extra Point 6 (*see* pages 31 and 35).

- Dip a cotton wool ball into the oil and squeeze it so that it's not dripping. Apply to your hair along the central parting. Continue to part your hair at regular intervals across the front of your head until you reach the tips of your ears, rubbing the oil onto the scalp as you go.

Replenish the cotton wool with oil as needed and repeat the process at the back of your head, until every inch of your scalp is covered lightly.

- Now use the balls of your fingers to manipulate your scalp and help loosen it. Apply as much pressure as is comfortable, going easily over tender spots. Most people find that they need to start very gently, pressing lightly with the fingers, progressively increasing the pressure so that the fingers are really working the scalp. Don't give up if it seems totally unyielding to begin with, it may take a few weeks before your scalp really starts to relax.

- Pay proper attention to the section at the base of the skull – which can become very tight – by circling your thumbs along the hairline with your fingers resting on the back of your head (*see* overleaf). Pour any remaining oil onto the central parting and rub vigorously. Run your fingers through your hair to disperse the oil.

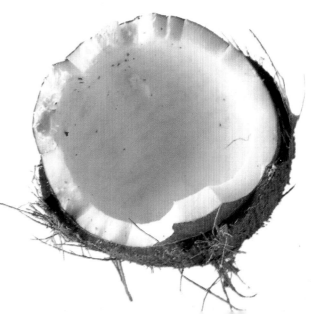

- Ideally the oil should be left on for a couple of hours – even better overnight. If you are in a hurry, apply the oil five to ten minutes before washing your hair. It will need two good lathers to remove all visible traces of the oil.

- Problem scalps need to be treated once a day for 12–14 weeks, decreasing to two to three times a week. After six months, you will be able to embark on a maintenance programme of weekly treatments. If you have psoriasis on your scalp, this regime will help to reduce the frequency of attacks, but resume daily treatment as soon as you feel an increase in the tightness and scaliness of your scalp.

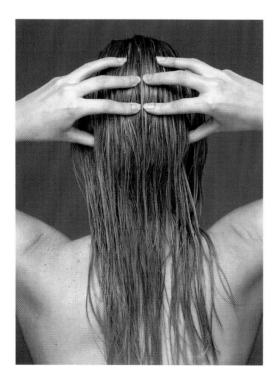

HAIR

Hair is an outgrowth of technically 'dead' cells originating in the living layer of the dermis. Each strand of hair consists of three parts: the outer cuticle, the central cortex and the inner medulla. The state of the cuticle – often compared to the scales on a fish – and the cortex are responsible for the condition of our hair. When the 'scales' lie flat, the surface of the hair is smooth and able to refract light, creating the sheen associated with healthy hair.

Like the skin, the hair has a natural protective coating of oil, produced in the follicle, which is of a slightly acidic nature. The one guiding principle when it comes to washing, treating and styling your hair is to avoid stripping your locks of this 'acid mantle' and roughing up the cuticle. This leaves the inside of the hair shaft vulnerable to damage and moisture evaporation, which results in weakened hair and problems such as split ends.

COMMON PROBLEMS

Hair Loss

Between 50 and 100 hairs can be lost naturally in the course of a single day. Hair loss and thinning hair, including the problem of male baldness, is generally caused by hormonal disruption – natural or induced – or hereditary factors beyond our control. High stress levels result in constricted circulation to the scalp, which is equivalent to cutting off the hair's food and water supply. Increased androgen levels and a disturbed menopause are other common triggers. In this situation, regular massage can help to make the most of the hair you have by boosting growth and conditioning hair to give the impression of bulk. If massage becomes a way of life at an early age, it is possible to inhibit an inherited tendency.

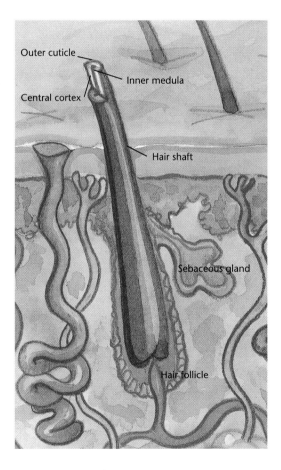

Cross section of hair shaft.

Outer cuticle

Inner medula

Central cortex

Hair shaft

Sebaceous gland

Hair follicle

Greying Hair

Like hair loss, greying hair is a powerful psychological issue. It occurs when insufficient melanin pigment is produced in the hair follicle to maintain our original hair colour. It is also sometimes linked to an iron deficiency. A huge number of us choose to colour our hair because we do not feel or want to look the age our changing hair colour suggests, or just because we feel like a change. If dyeing your hair, remember:

- Translucent dyes (rinses) allow the natural shading of each strand of hair to show through rather than imposing a blanket of colour.

- Highlights use bleach or a high-lift tint to give the hair a sun-dappled appearance, while lowlights introduce deeper glints. Both can be useful for creating an impression of volume in fine hair and camouflaging greying hair.

- Temporary and semi-permanent colours offer the chance to experiment without being stuck for too long with the result.

Provided that you take the trouble to protect and condition your hair and scalp (see above), I cannot see any downside in dyeing your hair. In fact, I am very much in favour of people learning how to colour their hair themselves, so that they can touch up new growth in between visits to the hairdresser.

If you do decide to colour your hair at home, make sure that you use a good, professional product and follow the instructions to the letter. Always wear gloves and apply a smear of Vaseline to protect the skin around your hairline. I am not a great fan of Henna, which has the unfortunate effect of tingeing grey hair red and, therefore, identifying the very hairs you are attempting to disguise.

WHAT TO DO

Feeding your Hair

Your hair, like the rest of your body, benefits from a healthy, balanced diet. Remember: extreme dieting deprives your hair of essential nutrients. Make the following a high priority:

- Lots of fresh fruit and vegetables (dark green leafy ones), eaten raw whenever possible.

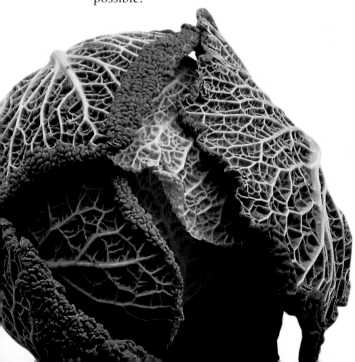

- Plenty of wholegrains and dried fruits.

- Protein taken regularly but in moderation.

- Eight to ten glasses of fresh water daily.

- Limited intake of refined carbohydrates, saturated fats, coffee, tea, sugar and salt.

Hair Washing

- Hair needs washing when it loses its 'bounce' and starts to look dull and lifeless. If your hair is oily or very fine, or you suffer from dandruff or psoriasis, you may not feel confident unless you give it a daily wash. Once your scalp is in peak condition, twice a week should be more than adequate.

- Detangle your hair before you wash it as wet hair is extremely fragile.

- Use a gentle, pH-balanced shampoo to preserve the hair's acid mantle.

- Squeeze the shampoo – just enough to generate a reasonable lather – into your palms before applying to your scalp and the roots of your hair. This is where it is most needed. Massage your scalp lightly all over with your fingertips while the shampoo is working, moving from the hairline towards the centre. Rinse and rinse until your hair 'squeaks'. A second shampoo will only be necessary if your hair is actually dirty.

- Use the smallest quantity of conditioner and comb it through your hair with your fingers, steering well clear of the roots.

If your hair is inclined to tangle, this is a good moment to comb it through very gently with a wide-toothed comb, starting at the ends and working slowly upwards. Rinse, rinse and rinse again.

- Cider vinegar (for dark hair and flaky/dandruff scalps) or lemon juice (for fair hair and greasy scalps) added to a basin of water as a final rinse will restore sheen and maintain the acid balance of your hair.

- Do not rub your hair – pat and squeeze it dry.

Blow-drying

- Wait until your hair is at least half dry before you attempt to style it.

- Do not use an appliance over 1200 watts and work with a diffuser attachment to spread the heat. Always keep the dryer moving, at a distance of about 6 inches from your hair. Dry from the roots to the ends.

- Dry your hair in the following order: back, sides, crown then front.

- Tip your head upside down to increase volume and experiment with root-lifting sprays.

- Dampen dry ends with a plant spray before styling to avoid heat damage.

- Allow your hair to dry naturally as often as possible, using your hands to create shape and lift the roots.

Extra Tips

- Wash your brushes and combs regularly with shampoo or detergent.

- Avoid brushes with synthetic bristles.

- The only remedy for split ends is to cut them off – they are impossible to 'mend'.

- Suncare – in India, the women use only their regular applications of oil to protect their hair from the hot sun. If you are oiling your hair at least once a week, it should be pretty well-screened from the damaging effect of the sun. Even so, covering your hair in intense sunlight is still advisable, particularly if your hair is coloured.

- Wear a close-fitting cap when swimming in a chlorinated pool. Coloured hair should also be protected from sea water.

- Zinc oxide in shampoo formulations acts as a useful three-way sunscreen, conditioner and anti-dandruff agent. Use in preference to dandruff shampoos containing coal tar, which has a drying effect on the hair shaft and is believed to be carcinogenic.

FOREHEAD

THE forehead is covered by a thin, wide band of muscle supported by a shallow layer of underlying tissue. This lack of 'padding', combined with a generous supply of nerve endings, makes the forehead particularly vulnerable to tension-damage below the surface. The skin on the forehead is more inclined to become congested too, as tension restricts the flow of blood and the removal of waste from the tissue. As a result, the normal shedding process of dead skin cells is disrupted, resulting in a thickening of the skin.

Smoking reduces the level of vitamin C available to the body essential for healthy collagen, as well as interfering with the supply of oxygen to the cells. An inadequate supply of protein in the diet will also adversely affect the production of new collagen and so, like smoking, lead to an increased tendency to premature lines and wrinkles.

The long-term effect of tension-damage on the forehead is a loss of elasticity in the connective tissue, which makes the skin more prone to line and wrinkle.

The more 'expressive' your forehead is, the greater the tendency to creasing and furrows.

Added to all this, the forehead rarely enjoys the same solicitous treatment as the rest of the face, so that the skin does not get the protection it needs.

The most common beauty problems affecting the forehead include:

PREMATURE LINES AND WRINKLES

Permanent creases are a sign that the collagen fibres – responsible for the resilience of the skin – have undergone a change which undermines their ability to erase the temporary lines made by habitual patterns of expression. It also points to a drop in the skin's oil and moisture levels – symptoms of stagnating circulation which may compound the problem (water is required to keep collagen pliable).

What to Do

- Boost your vitamin C count by including some fresh fruit and vegetables in every meal. Make sure that you are getting an adequate supply of protein.

A routine that *reduces*

fine lines and wrinkles

■ Try to stimulate the circulation to your forehead whenever you can, using small pinching movements. Increasing the blood supply to the forehead will nourish and help to repair the ailing tissue and help to bolster it against further damage. Once or twice a day will not be enough, you need to get be 'pinching' in every spare moment. Don't be too impatient for results, as it will probably be a few months before you see any marked improvement. After all, the lines did not appear overnight…

■ Be aware of when you are wrinkling your forehead or furrowing your brow and consciously relax the muscles to smooth out the skin.

Skincare & Make-up

■ Use a mild, oil-based cleanser or almond oil to avoid stripping the skin of its natural oil and moisture. Remove cleanser with a damp facial sponge.

■ Toning with an astringent preparation is not advised as it can just aggravate the condition. Use cold water or rosewater.

■ Use the Gentle Facial Exfoliator (*see* page 36) once a day for three weeks, then weekly, to combat the skin's tendency to accumulate dead cells.

■ Look out for a stabilizing face mask or make your own (*see* page 36). Use the mask on alternate days for the first three weeks, then once a week.

■ Use an oil-based foundation, applied with a damp sponge, then set with translucent loose powder.

CONGESTED AND SPOTTY SKIN

The forehead is a common area for spots to develop, particularly if the skin is oily (with overactive sebaceous glands) or overloaded with dead skin cells. The problem can be exacerbated by natural scalp oils and greasy cosmetics. There is also a tendency for this problem to flare up during periods of hormonal upheaval, such as pregnancy or puberty, when our sebaceous glands are at their most prolific.

Constipation and a clogged lymphatic system are often at the root of the problem. Don't forget that the skin is the body's main organ of elimination. When waste is not disposed of via the circulation or as a by-product of the digestive system, it may be excreted via the skin.

What to Do

■ Try to wear your hair off your face.

■ Avoid touching your forehead if you have an outbreak of spots. The oils from your fingers simply 'nourish' the spots as well as transporting bacteria to the area.

■ *Never* pick your spots if you want to prevent them becoming further infected and avoid scarring, which can be particularly conspicuous on the forehead.

- Avoid foods which seem to aggravate the problem and cut right back on your consumption of sugar, refined carbohydrates and saturated fats. A gentle detoxification programme, excluding wheat and dairy products from your diet for a three-month period (*see* page 156), or even fasting once a week, will reduce the potential irritants in the blood and calm the activities of the sebaceous glands. Eat plenty of fresh fruit and vegetables and fibre.

- For immediate help to control spots, use a spot treatment with anti-bacterial and antiseptic properties, such as a camphor-based preparation, to help control inflammation and cross-infection.

- Drink eight to ten glasses of water per day to flush out the system.

- *Always* remove your make-up before going to bed.

Skincare & Make-up

- Wash the affected area two or three times each day with a cleansing bar or a soap-free facial wash to remove skin 'grease' and control the spread of bacteria.

- Witch hazel mixed with a little water or saline solution is an effective toner.

Use a very small proportion of witch hazel on older skins, as it can have a drying effect.

- Use a light, oil-free moisturizer which will leave a protective film on the skin and stop infection going deeper into the follicle. Choose a non-comedogenic formulation – that is, one which will not block pores.

- Do not exfoliate the area as it stimulates the sebaceous glands in the dermis to produce more oil.

- Use the Cleansing Mask (*see* pages 36–37).

- Apply a turmeric and honey Healing Mask directly to spots (*see* pages 36–37) or use a camphor-based spot treatment.

- As for your make-up, use an oil-free, non-comedogenic foundation, such as a silicone-based product. Dab foundation on top of spots, then follow with a light overall application. Alternatively, concealer can be applied after foundation to camouflage blemishes. Dust with the finest covering of translucent powder.

IRREGULAR PIGMENTATION

Because of the forehead's thin tissue and prominent bones, the pigment cells lower down in the epidermis instantly leap to the skin's defence by discharging granules of protective melanin pigment if the forehead is left unprotected against the sun or subjected to excess rubbing or any other physical trauma. This can result in a mottled skin tone with some patches turning darker than others. Uneven pigmentation can also be caused by fluctuating female hormones and food allergens circulating in the bloodstream, as well as a rough-and-ready approach to skincare.

Try the following routines, but allow time for the pigmentation to readjust. You should notice some improvement after about three weeks, but persist until the problem is under control and then maintain the routine in a slightly reduced form to prevent a recurrence.

What to Do

- Always wear a sun block on your forehead. A hat with a deep brim will provide useful extra cover.

Skincare & Make-up

- Keep your routine as simple as possible. Avoid stimulation or irritation of melanin cells with harsh products and overzealous use of abrasive sponges.

- Cleanse with pH-balanced soap and water.

- Exfoliate daily for 6–12 weeks using a gentle formulation (*see* Exfoliator, page 36).

- Use a heavy moisturizer (oil-free if the skin is spotty as well), ideally with a built-in UV sunscreen. Alternatively, apply a fine sunscreen to the face after moisturizing – SPF (Sun Protection Factor) 15 is recommended year-round by dermatologists. Avoid any sun products containing oil of bergamot, as this accelerates the tanning process.

- No toner is needed.

- Foundation is important to help boost confidence. Try to wear a shade slightly darker than the pigmented area and apply all over the face, including ears, eyes and neck, to give uniform tone. There are many foundations on the market which contain a sunscreen too. Set with translucent loose powder.

DOWNY HAIR

Any hair visible on the upper part of the forehead is usually lighter and finer than other body hair and so of little consequence. However, sometimes this hair creates a shadowy effect, making the forehead look small and dark, particularly if the hairline is low.

What to Do

■ Preventative action is the best course. If a tendency to produce downy hair is apparent from an early age, rub the child's forehead *gently* with a towel after a bath. This helps to wear out the fine hairs which, after all, are only keratinized skin cells, without stimulating the follicle to become stronger. These downy hairs may well then disappear.

■ Alternatively, apply a freshly cut lemon to the forehead to make use of its natural bleaching agents.
　　Cut the lemon in half and rub it very gently over the hair and leave for five to seven minutes before rinsing off. Repeat whenever the darker new growth appears. Otherwise, seek professional advice about suitable methods of hair removal (*see* page 79).

Skincare & Make-up

■ Cleanse gently with pH-balanced soap and water so as not to overstimulate the area.

■ Moisturizer should be water-based to give as little nourishment as possible to hairs, and lightly massaged in.

■ No mask or toner is really required.

■ Avoid using foundation in this area, as it may show the hairs up more. If you tend to sweat a lot on your forehead, dust lightly with translucent loose powder, as this absorbs water.

O NE of our most beautiful and individual features, our eyes reflect our vitality, emotions and general state of health. How we use them is also important: bright eyes and immediate eye contact impart directness and confidence; downcast eyes suggest timidity and low self-esteem.

While the eyes themselves are fairly robust, the skin around the eyes is particularly thin and delicate. Not as firmly attached to the underlying muscle and bone as the skin in other parts of the face, it is more inclined to stretch and become loose. For this reason, special care should be taken not to pull or drag the skin when applying or removing make-up, as this can hasten the arrival of premature wrinkles.

Mainly serviced by lymphatic vessels, which do not have the efficient pumping mechanism of the heart to rely on, the eye tissue is prone to stagnation. This is especially likely to happen when the lymphatic fluid is thicker due to the chemical changes that occur just before a period.

Stagnation stops the eyes looking clear and is the root cause of many conditions affecting the eyelids.

The underlying tissue is also poorly supplied with sebaceous glands, hence the need for good lubrication and nourishment in the eye area. Despite the faith placed in cosmetic eye creams, the surest way to noursh the skin and look after the health of your eyes is by eating well (see page 156) and by giving the circulation a regular helping hand. Eyes also flourish on a simple regime of rest, exercise and natural light. They do not take well to excessive smoking or alcohol.

COMMON PROBLEMS

Puffy Eyes

Lack of sleep (or sometimes too much sleep) and sensitivity to certain skin and make-up products are the most common causes of puffy eyes, although sluggish circulation, causing stagnation and waterlogged tissue around the eyes, can sometimes play a part. Puffy eyes may also indicate a thyroid problem or signal constipation.

Bright eyes *reflect* your

body's good health

Dark Circles

Some people are definitely more prone to the 'panda eye' syndrome than others. This can be brought on by a shortage of sleep, poor circulation or poor elimination, all of which cause the blood to acquire a bluish tinge and encourage pigments and waste to settle in the delicate tissue around the eye.

Shadows are more apparent when the skin is thin or fair, as the underlying blood vessels are more visible. However, in darker skins, where the tendency to pigment is greater, irritating waste deposits which 'traumatize' the skin around the eyes are more inclined to trigger the release of protective melanin granules, potentially causing deeper discoloration.

Unless it is properly addressed, the problem can become deep-seated. Once it reaches this stage, even intensive therapy cannot eradicate the circles, although they may become two or three shades lighter as the stagnation is dispersed and the supporting tissue becomes healthier.

Dark circles may also occur as a result of kidney problems, food intolerance or various nutritional deficiencies, including iron, vitamin C and vitamin B$_{12}$.

Tired Eyes

Sleep deprivation is almost guaranteed to make your eyes look dull and lifeless. Try to catch up on lost hours with a few early nights (advancing your bedtime by

To preserve your eyes and your eyesight, eat plenty of fruit and vegetables, poultry, fish, nuts, wholegrains, seeds and their oils. Opt for orange-coloured fruits and vegetables, dark green, leafy vegetables and avocados whenever possible. Limit your consumption of saturated animal fat to the minimum.

an hour or more pays dividends). Otherwise, a cold compress (a cotton wool pad soaked in cold water) will relieve and rest tired eyes by reducing the blood flow to the area. It will also help to remove any toxic build-up in eye muscles and tissue. Leave in place for 10–15 minutes.

Reading or writing without adequate light or concentrating on close work for lengthy periods can make eyes unreasonably tired, causing vision to blur and, eventually, to deteriorate. It is therefore essential that we rest them regularly during periods of intensive eye work (try the palming exercise described on page 60). Staring at a VDU for hours on end is particularly wearing on the eyes and needs to be punctuated by a 10 minute break every couple of hours.

Droopy Eyes

This is caused by a lack of muscle tone in the upper eyelid, combined with the downward force of gravity. The circular eye muscle, responsible for opening and closing the eye, is extremely delicate. However, if massaged regularly over a period of time, it is possible to regain some degree of tone. The first exercise described on page 60 will also help to condition the muscle.

Crêpey Eyelids

Smooth eye contours desert us all at some point, but many eyelids turn crêpey (intensely lined and wrinkled) before their time because they are constantly exposed to irritants contained in cosmetics and skincare products.

Circulation and diet also have an impact on the texture of the skin around the eyes, in so far as they affect the production of collagen (which reinforces the tissue), and the condition of the muscle (which has the capacity to hold the skin taut).

Dry Skin

Dehydrated skin around the eyes is usually attributed to the small number of sebaceous glands in the area and the falling moisture level of the skin as we age. Harsh cleansing products or unsuitable make-up can aggravate the problem. Overstimulation can also disrupt the activities of the sebaceous glands. Choose any eye preparations with great care and give the eyes a regular therapy (*see* page 12). If you ignore the problem, the skin tone may also become darker.

Crow's Feet

We all develop these natural lines of expression over time, but if the skin around the eyes is well-moisturized, they simply add to the character of the face. When the skin is allowed to become dry, however, these lines which radiate from the outer corner of our eyes can become deeply etched, which can age the face prematurely.

Certain habitual patterns of facial expression encourage crow's feet. They tend to be more pronounced in smokers, for example, who are constantly squinting to avoid the smoke they produce. Sun damage accelerates the formation of such facial lines.

WHAT TO DO

■ A slice of cucumber placed on each eyelid for up to 15 minutes is very soothing. Cucumber has a high mineral and water content which is therapeutic for the eyes. The juice also makes a nourishing eye drop.

■ Always wear sunglasses (with ultraviolet or UV *and* infrared ray protection) in bright sunlight and to help your eyes acclimatize to a sudden increase in light. Remember, however, that your eyes, like the rest of your body, suffer if they are starved of natural light, so try to spend some time outside every day and allow your eyes to go unshaded from time to time in gentle sunlight.

Exercise

For lasting results, carry out the lymphatic draining exercise on page 12 night and morning. It will only add a few seconds to your cleansing routine.

Performed regularly, the following exercises will keep eyes clear and whites white. They can also help to maintain perfect vision and improve failing sight. Practise them once a day. I do them in the loo, although bath time is a good moment too.

For firm, taut eyelids:

- Shut both eyelids tightly so that you feel the squeezing effect on the eyes. Maintain this pressure for a count of 12. Relax the eyelids. Rest the eyes for a moment by keeping them lightly closed. Repeat five times.

To strengthen the different muscles of the eye:

- Keeping your head still, move your eyes as far to the right as you can without straining them. Blink, then do the same to the left. Blink and repeat six times on each side. Rest your eyes by keeping them lightly closed for a count of 20.

- Keeping your head still, raise your eyes as high as you can. Blink once, then lower your eyes as far as you can. Blink again and repeat the sequence six times. Now rest your eyes.

- Keeping your head still, look up towards your right eyebrow. Blink and look down towards your left earlobe. Repeat the sequence six times, then rest the eyes for a count of 20. Now do the left eyebrow and the right earlobe. Rest the eyes.

'Palming' is a very effective way to rest and relax tired or strained eyes, as the palms create the condition of total darkness the eyes require to recuperate.

- Sit with your elbows resting on a table or on the floor with your back against a wall and your elbows propped on raised knees.

- Close your eyes and cover them completely, with the palms of your hands slightly cupped and your fingers resting on the front of your head. Make sure that you are not pressing on your eyeballs. Remain in this position for several minutes, breathing slowly and deeply.

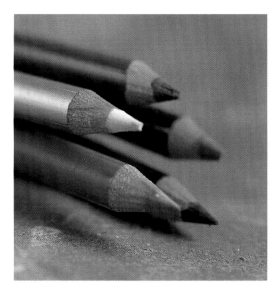

SKINCARE

Apart from treating your eyes gently, the principle of good eye care is to use the bare minimum and stick to natural products.

There is no end of specially targeted eye creams and gels available, a number of which are remarkably effective in tightening and 'plumping' the skin, apparently eradicating fine lines. However, the effects produced by this cosmetic approach are only temporary and the actual state of the eye tissue is unchanged. If your eyes are sensitive, look out for the terms 'hypoallergenic' and 'allergy-tested'. Eczema sufferers should screen ingredients lists for possible sensitizers. Some further tips:

■ Make your own nourishing Eye Mask (*see* page 37).

■ Look for a moisturizer with a built-in sunscreen for daytime use, especially if you are fair-skinned or have a tendency to develop shadows around the eyes.

■ Never use a toner on the eyes. Simply splash your eyes with cold water after cleansing, which will also invigorate the circulation.

■ Almond oil, one of the most gentle and versatile skincare tools, is perfect for dissolving eye make-up and cleansing the eye area. If you wear a lot of eye make-up, cleanse twice, removing the excess oil by sweeping across the skin gently with a damp, natural sponge or cotton wool pad. Avoid seepage into the corner of the eye by using no more than the quantity required to lubricate your strokes. This oil also makes a nourishing base (blot the excess with a tissue to prevent your make-up from smearing). Alternatively, use a light, water-based moisturizer.

People are brainwashed into over-tending the eyes, which can do as much damage as total neglect. Whatever you do, don't fall into the trap of slathering your eyes with a super-rich cream to replace lost moisture and restore suppleness, as this will simply overtax the delicate eye tissue and do nothing to enhance your eyes.

MAKE-UP

Eyes provide the perfect canvas for make-up and offer the potential for creating many effects. Remember, however: too much make-up, badly applied, can distract and detract from the eyes instead of flattering them.

The value of eye make-up is that it can subtly emphasize individual qualities while playing down any imperfections. Most of us would like to be able to achieve maximum impact with a few deft strokes before we emerge to start the day or in preparation for an evening out. The following suggestions may help.

■ Make-up around the eyes should be applied gently and evenly, on top of a light foundation and powder base. Make sure that the foundation covers the temples – without straying into the hairline – and both the upper and

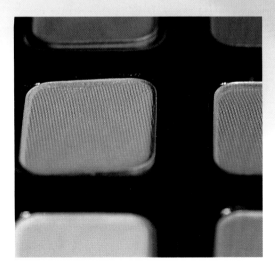

lower eyelids. Use a creamy concealer to camouflage dark circles and any shadows around the eyes and pat gently with the pad of your middle finger to blend. Finish with a fine application of translucent powder.

■ The simplest way to add definition to your eyes is with an eye pencil. Black tends to suit dark-eyed, dark-skinned women best, whereas brown and charcoal are more neutral, versatile shades which work with a range of complexions and eye colours. Draw the line as close to your eyelashes as possible, top and bottom – it is up to you whether you start at the inner corner of the eye or a little way out – and gently smudge it if you wish to soften the effect (some pencils have a sponge on the end for this purpose). It may be enough to line the upper lid only or you might achieve the effect you want with an additional fine line of eyeshadow.

■ Powder eyeshadow is the most popular choice (contact lens wearers should look for flake-resistant varieties). Steer clear of anything too obviously pearly or matt. Again, try to stick to a neutral palette (earth tones, smoky greys and browns, violets and heathery shades), as these complement most eye colours and can be blended to create a natural effect. Apply colour thinly and gradually, darkest along the lid and at the outer corner of the eyes.

■ Mascara accentuates and 'opens up' the eyes, as well as adding a touch of glamour. To apply successfully, look down into a mirror and brush the lashes through slowly, from roots to tips. Start with the top side, then the underside of the upper lashes. Rest the brush on the outside of the lower lashes to give a light covering. Apply two or three thin coats for best results – the final coat may be just to emphasize outer tips. Separate any clogged lashes with an eyelash comb.

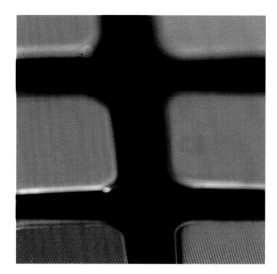

Semi-permanent Make-up

With this form of cosmetic tattooing, pigments are implanted between the roots of the eyelashes or eyebrows to create an impression of colour and thickness. It can be done on both upper and lower lids as well as on the eyebrows and gives the eyes a naturally made-up look, without being artificial. It is also an effective way of both filling in gaps when the eyebrows have been over-plucked or growth is sparse and of camouflaging any birth marks or scar tissue, for example.

This – usually corrective – treatment may be worth considering if, for some reason such as failing eyesight, applying make-up is difficult for you to do. Make sure that you have a patch test done first and remember that you can always ask the practitioner to stop at any moment, so you can see the effect.

Perming Lashes

Eyelash perming is a very popular technique in the East. I learnt it while I was in Hong Kong and was surprised and impressed at the way it can enhance the eyes. The alternative is to use eyelash curlers, but the effects are short-lived (an eyelash perm can last up to three months) and lashes can be weakened by frequent use. If you do want to experiment with curlers, avoid the cheapest metal ones and remember to curl lashes *before* you apply mascara.

PLUCKING BROWS

Some people are lucky enough to be born with shapely, tidy eyebrows. Most of us, however, have our work cut out trying to tame unruly brows and keep growth under control. Here are a few practical tips which may make the task a little easier.

■ The most natural and flattering eyebrow shape is an arc with its highest point above the outside of the iris (*see* page 65). Start by removing hairs from the inner edge and the bridge of the nose. Now prune the centre and outer edge, allowing the line to taper gradually to nothing. To find out where the brow should end, imagine a line connecting the outside of your nostril with the outer corner of your eye and extending out to your brow. Finally, pull out any stray hairs below the brows. The less you pluck, the easier it is to maintain the shape. Over-plucking may leave you with permanently sparse brows.

■ If you are sensitive to pain, pull gently upwards on the outside edge of your eyebrow while you pluck. Tolerance of pain also appears to be reduced during menstruation, so delay your reshaping job until mid-cycle if your threshold is low.

■ Troublesome eyebrows it is worth entrusting to a professional therapist, who will either pluck them into shape or use a technique called 'threading'. This is an ancient practice which involves tightening a piece of fine, cotton thread around each hair to remove it. If done properly, every hair

Tinting Brows and Lashes

If your eyebrows are too fair for your liking, have them tinted a darker shade. This helps to frame the eyes and saves having to achieve the effect with make-up. Avoid going too dark, however, as you may end up looking like a pantomime villain! Eyelashes also look more glossy and striking when they have been tinted.

Tints are usually vegetable-based and rarely damage the hairs. If anything, they tend to nourish the follicle, strengthening growth. Tinting should be repeated every six weeks or so. Although there are kits for home dyeing, it is safer to have it done professionally and the effect is longer-lasting because stronger preparations can be used. Brushing eyebrows with an almost empty mascara brush is another way of creating a stronger brow line.

is removed at the same tension from the root. This weakens the hair growth and removes the shadowy effect on the brows. The advantages of this method are minimum regrowth and no damage to the follicles.

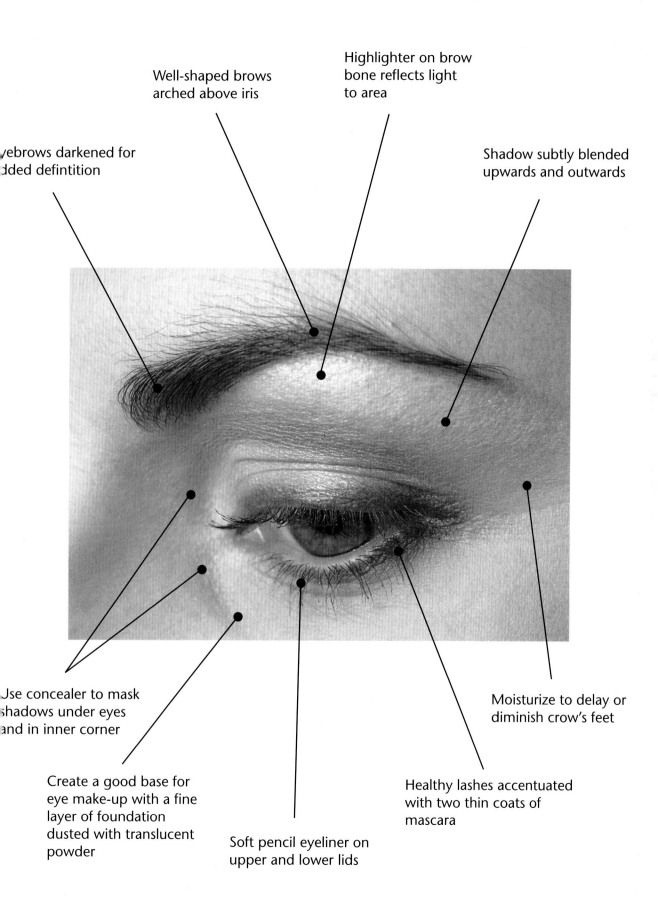

Well-shaped brows
arched above iris

Highlighter on brow
bone reflects light
to area

Shadow subtly blended
upwards and outwards

yebrows darkened for
dded defintition

Use concealer to mask
shadows under eyes
and in inner corner

Create a good base for
eye make-up with a fine
layer of foundation
dusted with translucent
powder

Soft pencil eyeliner on
upper and lower lids

Healthy lashes accentuated
with two thin coats of
mascara

Moisturize to delay or
diminish crow's feet

CHEEKS

THE cheeks consist of several thin muscles stretched across a bony frame (*see* page 170). While the structure and scale of the cheeks is determined by the shape and size of the bones underneath, the muscle fibres are responsible for creating their contours – firm or otherwise. Beneath the muscle lies a series of hollow spaces which are favourite spots for waste, fat and lymph to collect. When there is an accumulation of these deposits, the natural shape of the cheeks becomes distorted.

Our complexion – generally judged from the skin on the cheeks – serves as a barometer for our inner health. When the body is in balance, the texture of the skin can be as smooth and fine as the proverbial peach, and the skin tone warm and even. When the internal harmony of the body

The colouring of our cheeks is strongly influenced by the circulation. Lost bloom cannot therefore be restored simply by slapping on extra moisturizer. When bright red, oxygen-rich blood is whooshing through the capillaries, our cheeks positively glow. When our oxygen levels are low and the circulation sluggish, however, we look pale and washed out. Vigorous circulation in the facial area also helps to keep the complexion clear and maintain the condition of the muscles.

is disturbed by hormonal activity, stress, diet, constipation or illness, our cheeks usually suffer.

While we cannot prevent the changes that occur as part of the ageing process, we can certainly ensure that we do not prejudice the health and beauty of our cheeks by our own ignorance.

Common problems concerning the cheeks include:

A skincare programme to

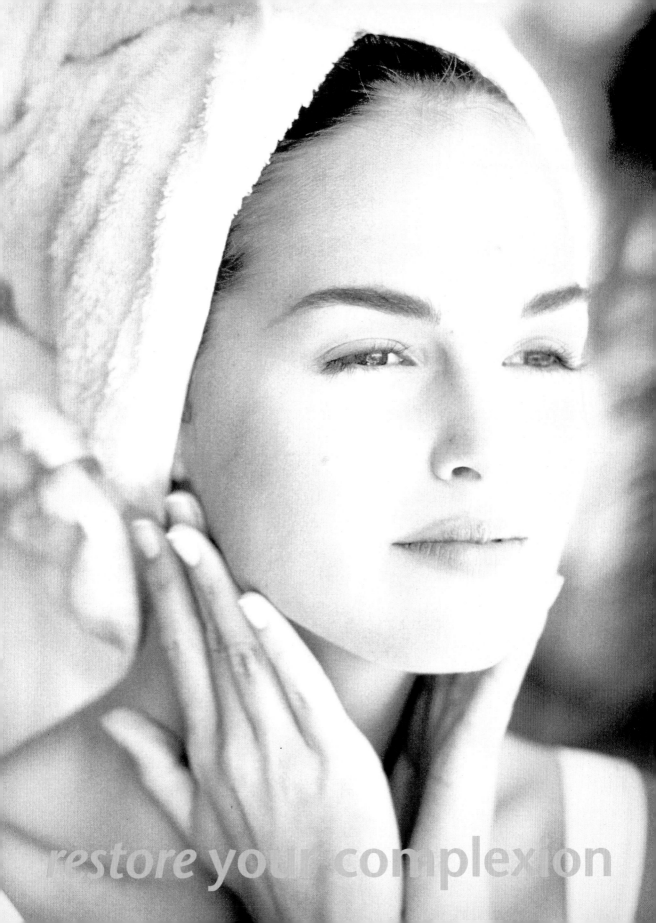

restore your complexion

PODGY CHEEKS

An indication of poor circulation and, usually, excess weight. Blood and lymph leave too much waste and unwelcome fat in the tissue beneath the thin cheek muscle, which results in the cheeks becoming distended. There may be a puffy quality to the cheeks if there is a lot of fluid being held in the cheeks. It is also not uncommon for the cheeks to become fuller and heavier at the time of the menopause. Digestive problems are another possible cause.

Skincare

When the cheeks are full, the skin is more stretched and, therefore, more easily irritated. It is important to avoid this, as a skin reaction could interfere with the firming and toning process.

- Use a water-based cleanser or a pH-balanced soap and remove with a damp, natural sponge or cotton wool pad.

- Moisturize with almond oil, which can then be gently massaged into the cheeks using the palms of your hands. Remove excess oil with a tissue and apply a water-based moisturizer if you need to. Otherwise, simply leave your skin as it is, protected by a film of almond oil.

- Use the Firming Mask (*see* page 37) once a week.

What to Do

Exercise

Get into the habit of carrying out the following 'pinch and drain' routine regularly if you have a tendency to put on weight on your face. Remember: a slim face will make you feel slimmer all over. The technique will galvanize circulation and improve muscle tone, as well as encouraging drainage. It will also help to clear the sinuses, which can become slightly compressed when the cheeks are heavy.

- Using your thumbs to apply pressure to the undersides of your cheekbones, pinch the flesh on the top of the cheeks with your index finger. Still sustaining the pressure, glide your thumbs a little further along the bone and pinch again. Repeat until you reach the point where the cheekbones and jaw hinges meet.

- Using your index finger, apply even pressure at this point for a count of 10. Release and repeat three times. Do this twice a day to drain the cheeks, reducing the frequency as they start to become firm.

DROOPY CHEEKS

We are all prepared for our cheeks to drop with the passing of the years, but there are other reasons why cheeks may sag suddenly and dramatically. If they are overburdened by excess bulk for too long (*see* above), the muscle tone will gradually weaken under the strain. The problem may equally be caused by weight-loss as a result of crash dieting, when the face seems to be the first place to emulsify its stores of fat. Damage caused by chronic acne can also undermine the support structure beneath the cheeks. Plastic surgery may be required to correct serious cases.

What to Do

■ Massage your cheekbones and the underlying tissue regularly using the pinch and drain method described on page 68.

Skincare

See advice for Podgy Cheeks, page 68.

CONGESTED AND SPOTTY SKIN

When the circulation in the cheek area is sluggish, the hair follicles become congested with oil and dead skin cells and toxins start to settle in the spaces beneath the cheek muscles. This alters the pH balance of the skin, allowing blocked follicles to become infected and inflamed by bacteria that normally live harmlessly on the skin. Whiteheads occur when the sticky 'plug' that is blocking the follicle is enclosed by dead skin cells which have accumulated on the surface of the skin.

> If you embark on a programme of weight-loss, make sure that you do so with the help of a balanced, health-promoting eating plan (*see* page 161). It is essential to aim for a slow, gradual weight-loss which allows time for the skin tone to improve as the underlying elastic tissue takes in the slack.

What to Do

■ Use the pinch and drain method described earlier. Once the circulation is a little brisker, it will relieve congestion in the follicles and help to clear the toxins that have become trapped in the area.

■ Help to draw out these toxins via the skin with the Healing Mask (*see* page 36).

Skincare

See advice in the relevant Forehead section, page 53.

EXCESS HAIR

We all have a fine covering of downy hair on our faces, which may be more obvious when the skin and hair colour is darker. Generally it only becomes a problem if hairs are bristly or pigmented as a result of hormonal imbalances which reach their peak during adolescence and the menopause.

Unsuitable skincare products and routines are as much to blame for excess hair problems as misguided attempts at removing the offending hair. These can both 'traumatize' the hair follicles, which results in the emergency delivery of blood by the circulatory system containing 'food parcels' for the follicle. With this additional nourishment, the follicle goes on to produce a stronger hair.

What to Do

Prevention is better than cure. If a child has a tendency to facial hair, encourage *gentle* rubbing with a face cloth as part of the morning wash or bathtime routine. Adults should employ the same technique, while sticking to the skincare principles outlined below.

Electrolysis

If the hair has already been tampered with, the distorted follicles may have started to produce stronger hair with stronger pigments. In this situation, professional treatment is advisable. Before you embark on electrolysis, however, it is important to establish that your skin is fit enough to take the treatment (*see also* page 77). Invasive, needle-based methods can result in the formation of scar tissue if the skin is not sufficiently supple, so you may prefer to try one of the non-invasive methods of electrolysis.

I strongly recommend the American TE (Transdermal Electrolysis) system. Permanent and painless, there is also no risk of scarring. This method uses a probe, rather than a needle or tweezers, immersed in a special ionized gel to transmit a galvanic current through the skin to the hair follicles. As a result, a chemical reaction occurs in the follicle which destroys the root. Hair scanning is another gentle, pain-free, non-invasive option which works through a high-intensity radio frequency and is suitable for hypersensitive skin types.

If the hair growth seems abnormal, it might be helpful to have a hormonal check to establish the cause and the need for permanent hair removal.

Skincare

You need to follow a skincare routine which does not irritate or stimulate your skin. As mentioned earlier, any additional nourishment, via creams or improved blood flow to the follicles, will strengthen the hair growth, making the hair more substantial and darker in pigment.

- Use the Lemon-based Mask (*see* page 37) and repeat once a month, or when darker regrowth appears.

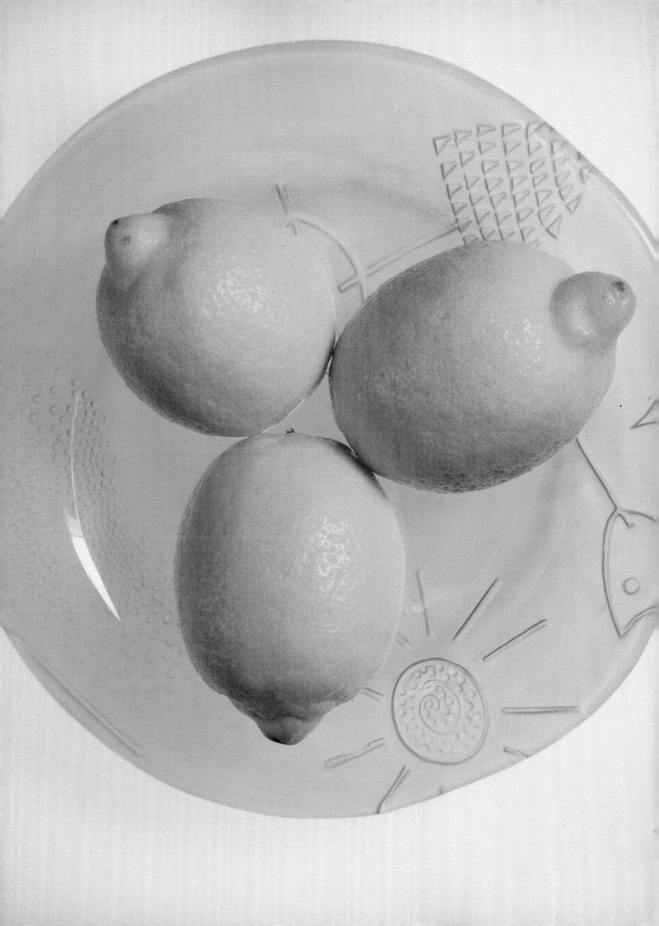

- Tone with rosewater as this has a calming effect.

- Use a very light moisturizer.

- Cleanse gently with pH-balanced soap and water or a very mild cleanser.

IRREGULAR PIGMENTATION

Some women are prone to develop darker patches of skin on the face as a result of the hormonal changes which take place during pregnancy, the menopause and while taking the contraceptive pill. The problem occurs most commonly on the cheeks and around the mouth and spots may merge, forming the so-called 'mask of pregnancy' or chloasma. This usually disperses of its own accord in a three to six month period after the baby is born. Sometimes the skin just appears tanned and freckles a little darker.

Irregular pigmentation on the face may also follow an outbreak of acne or eczema and can even be brought on by overzealous exfoliation. Liver spots, which are a fairly common feature of mature skin, are caused by clusters of pigment triggered by exposure to ultraviolet rays. They may also be linked to a vitamin B-complex deficiency.

What to Do

- Hormonally related pigmentation should correct itself, but if the patches do not disappear within six months, see your GP to check hormone levels. If the problem persists, it might be worth considering professional treatment to stimulate circulation to the basal layer of the skin, which can help to disperse the pigment.

- As soon as you notice pigmentation marks developing on your cheeks, start wearing a high-protection sunscreen at all times. Apply a sun block if your cheeks are going to be exposed to intense sunlight.

- A vitamin B-complex supplement, supported by a balanced diet, may help to clear liver spots.

Skincare

See advice in the relevant Forehead section, page 52.

DRY CHEEKS (WITH COMBINATION SKIN)

With so-called combination skin, cheeks have a tendency to dryness, while the 'T' zone (forehead, nose and chin) remains oily. To bring nourishment to the deprived cheek area, gentle stimulation is needed. For the best results, follow different, relevant skincare routines for the central oily panel and the cheeks.

What to Do

■ Pinch and drain the cheek area to brighten up the complexion (*see* page 68).

■ Beware of overstimulating the central panel as this will increase the activities of the sebaceous glands.

■ As a preventative measure, avoid hot, spicy food and excessive consumption of alcohol. These can have a sensitizing effect on fragile blood capillaries in the cheeks.

■ Drink eight to ten glasses of water per day.

Skincare

■ A gentle, cream-based cleanser should be applied to the cheeks and washed off with a damp, natural sponge or cotton wool pad.

■ Moisturize separately with an oil-based moisturizer.

■ Apply the Nourishing Cheek Face Mask (*see* page 37). This will help loosen dead cells enabling healthy, new ones to take their place.

MAKE-UP

■ Match skin tone with foundation. If the skin on your cheeks is dry, look for a formulation with a creamy texture. An oil-free (ideally, non-comedogenic) foundation or a compact foundation/ powder is more suitable for oily skin and enlarged pores. For a more natural look, or if there is a lot of facial hair, try one of the tinted moisturizers available. A light mousse-based foundation works well on skin with eczema.

■ Using downwards strokes, apply foundation all over the face using a damp make-up sponge or just blend into areas of higher colour with your fingers to even up skin tone. If you are applying foundation darker than your natural skin tone for camouflage purposes, don't forget to include neck, ears and nostrils as well.

■ Concealers are very effective in covering blemishes and small areas of discoloration. Apply a little at a time on top of foundation and blend well. If pigmentation is more widespread, choose a foundation which is a shade darker than the pigmented area. This is where mixing skills using two different foundations come in useful.

■ If a natural glow is all you are after, a touch of cream blusher applied to well-moisturized cheeks will do the trick.

■ Good cheekbones are definitely worth emphasizing. Load up a proper blusher brush with a small amount of colour and blow off the excess. Sweep the brush across your cheekbones in the direction of – but short of – the hairline. Alternatively, swirl a bushy brush in circles on the apples of your cheeks to make pale cheeks look healthy.

■ Tie in your blusher with your lipstick – if your lip colour is 'cool', your blusher colour should be too.

■ Elaborate contouring is best left to the professionals as it is prone to misfire, leaving you – instead of looking like a hollow-cheeked starlet – with a series of conspicuous stripes running across your face. However, if you have full cheeks, try using a light application of a powder a shade darker than your foundation (sometimes called 'faceshaper') on the underside of cheekbones, blended out towards the ears, as this does add definition.

■ Foundation looks more finished when set with a very light dusting of loose translucent powder. Tip a small quantity into the palm of your hand, soak some up with a velours puff or cotton wool pad, then apply. Remove any excess with a large brush or a clean pad. Alternatively, use a brush to apply powder, having first blown off any excess. Pressed powder is a more practical choice when you are on the move.

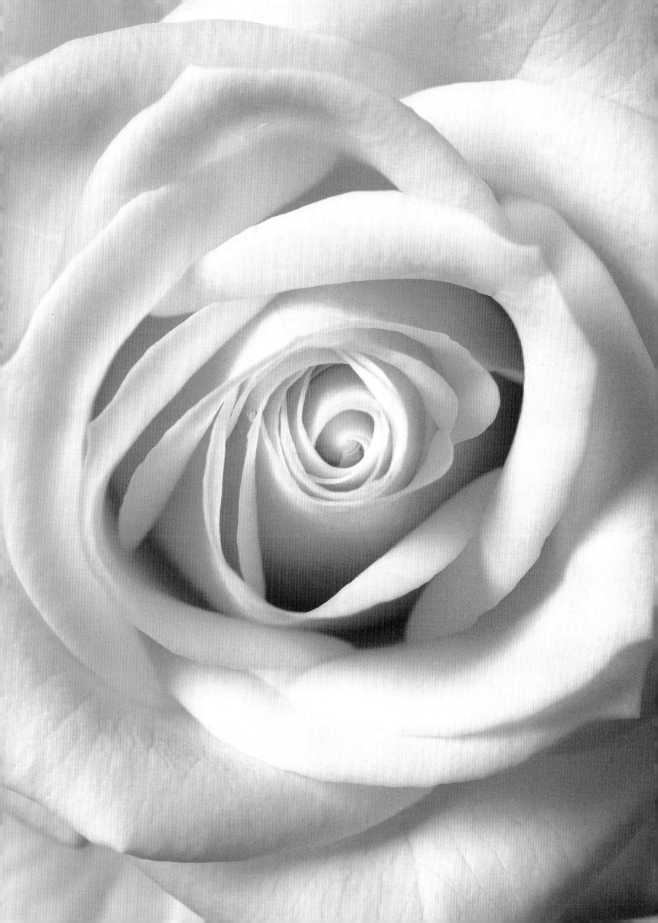

Your mouth is your

MOUTH

OUR mouth is the most sensual feature of our face, both from the point of view of our appearance and the sensations it enables us to experience. The texture and condition of our lips contribute as much as the overall shape and contours of our mouth to its allure. A deft hand with the right lipstick and a healthy set of teeth are all that is required to complete the picture.

We express our pleasure and our displeasure via our mouths. We talk about a 'winning' smile and we all respond to a smiling face. It is worth noting that, when our faces are in repose, they can become set in an unconscious grimace, which makes us look permanently sour and grumpy. Break this habit by becoming aware of your facial expression and consciously altering it.

Our lips are covered on the outside by a thin layer of skin and on the inside by virtually transparent mucous membranes, and are very easily damaged. Unlike most of the skin on the body, they do not have any melanin pigments to protect them. A sunscreen in summer and a barrier cream in winter are therefore vital to keep our lips smooth and soft.

Common problems I encounter affecting the lips include:

LINES ON THE UPPER LIP

Premature lines and wrinkles on the upper lip sometimes result from damage to the tissue caused by the treatment of superfluous hair. Hair removing and bleaching creams contain strong chemicals which can act as a powerful irritant, particularly to sensitive skin, hence the importance of doing a patch test on the skin in advance. If you feel an itching sensation or your skin becomes red or inflamed after applying one of these, it is a clear sign that it is doing harm. Remove it immediately and do not attempt to use it again.

Electrolysis treatment should also be embarked upon with some caution since this process works by attracting moisture from nearby cells to create a chemical reaction which destroys the hair follicle. If electrolysis is carried out when the moisture level of the skin is depleted, it can hasten the degeneration process in the supporting tissue. Subsequent neglect of areas of electrolysed skin, allowing them to become dehydrated, can have similar consequences.

Pucker lines and wrinkles on the upper lip come early to heavy smokers, due to the repeated movements of the mouth involved in the action of smoking

most *sensual* feature

and the reduced levels of oxygen and collagen that nicotine causes. This can add years to your face, as can the tendency to pout, which a lot of people do without realizing it. Sun damage is another major culprit.

What to Do

■ Twitching your nose is an effective way of mobilizing the muscles in the middle of the face. The idea is to make small up-and-down movements without creating too many creases over the bridge. If you practise while looking in a mirror, you will see how it activates the cheek area and the skin between the nose and mouth.

■ Almond oil applied to your lips and the skin around your mouth will help to keep the area supple.

Exercise
I very much believe in exercise to strengthen the muscles around the mouth and improve the underlying circulation. Once the circulation is normalized, damaged cells receive more nourishment to assist the repair process and a regular supply of moisture. Make a point of doing this exercise whenever you have a spare moment and you could feel a firming effect in as little as a week.

■ Close your mouth and inflate the skin above the upper lip and on either side of the mouth, while you continue to breathe through your nose (*see* right).

■ Hold for a count of 10 and then repeat 10 times.

■ You must keep your upper lip smooth and relaxed throughout – it may help to position one finger above each corner of your mouth to hold the skin in place.

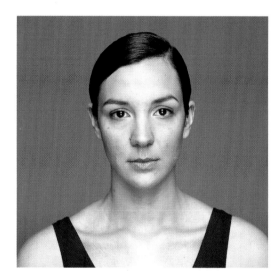

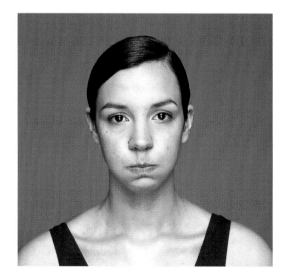

HAIR ON THE UPPER LIP

This problem is fairly common, especially for dark-haired women. It is unwise to try to tackle the problem with depilatory creams and bleaches for the reasons outlined above (*see* page 77), or to experiment with home waxing, as you risk distorting the follicles, which could add to the problem and make any damage harder to rectify. There are, however, several methods of permanent hair removal which are safe and effective in the hands of a reliable practitioner.

What to Do

■ If the problem is causing distress, I recommend threading (*see* page 64) initially to clear the area. The choice is then between electrolysis using the faster, direct current method or the gentler, galvanic method (*see* page 70). This will depend on state of the skin and diameter of the hair. With very sensitive skin conditions such as psoriasis, opt for a system which uses gel rather than a needle to destroy the follicle.

While it is heartening to know that facial hair can be eliminated without disfiguring side effects, I remain convinced that prevention is by far the best approach to the problem. From the earliest infancy girls should be encouraged to rub the affected skin *gently* with a towel/face cloth or to bleach with lemon juice.

BLACKHEADS

Clogged pores and blackheads around the outer edge of the lips, caused by sluggish circulation, are very common. If the underlying problem is not addressed, pores become stretched and may remain permanently open. Any attempts to squeeze blackheads or to remove them with a metal implement can leave small scars which break up your lipline.

What to Do

■ Try light exfoliation (*see* Gentle Facial Exfoliator, page 36) every day until you see an improvement. This will decongest the area.

■ Follow with the Cleansing Mask (*see* page 36).

DEHYDRATED AND CRACKED LIPS

The skin on our lips becomes dehydrated when the natural oils which help to keep it supple are reduced or removed. If the moisture is not replenished, and the lips are not protected by a balm or cream, they can become flaky and crack. This is both uncomfortable and unsightly. The most common causes of dehydration are extreme weather conditions, an allergic reaction to cosmetics or, when the corners of the mouth are affected, a B-vitamin deficiency. Eczema and local infections also have a drying effect on the upper layers of the skin on our lips.

What to Do

- Resist the natural desire to lick dry lips for temporary relief as this only makes them dryer still.

- I am a great believer in Vaseline as a protection for the lips. Apply to dehydrated or cracked lips several times a day.

SKINCARE & MAKE-UP

- The skin above your upper lip needs to be treated gently and moisturized generously. If your skin is sensitive, use almond oil for both purposes.

> Face cloths are very useful for sweeping away dead skin cells and gingering up the circulation in this area without subjecting your skin to further irritation.

- Once you have given your moisturizer a chance to sink in, apply a light wash of foundation with a damp sponge and set with a touch of powder. If you have darker blotches of skin, use a lighter foundation or concealer beneath the powder as a camouflage.

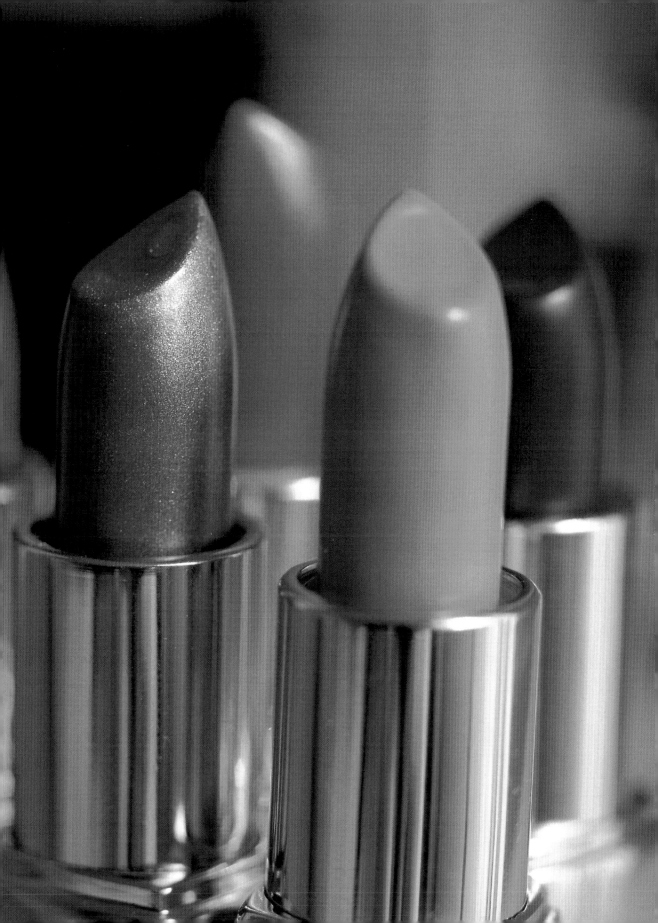

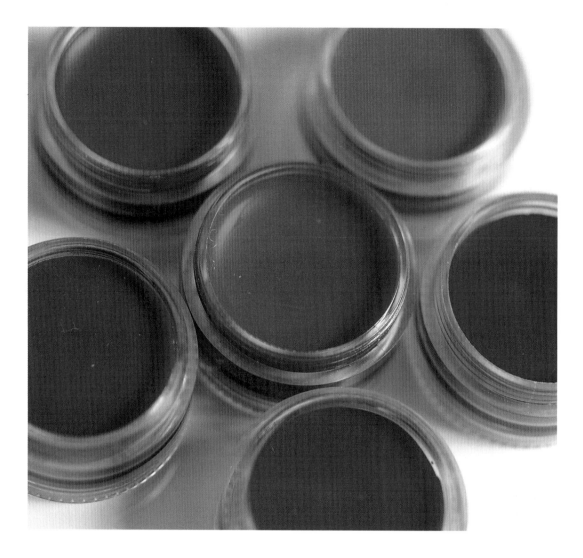

■ Lips need to be screened from potentially damaging ultraviolet rays and harsh winter weather, so look out for lipsticks with SPFs and other nourishing ingredients.

■ To boost the circulation and lift dead skin, massage your lips from time to time with a soft toothbrush.

■ Semi-permanent pigments can be injected around the lips to fill in a broken lipline or camouflage scarring or other damage. It is also an effective way to extend an excessively narrow upper lip. A highly skilled practitioner will mix the pigments to match your natural lip colour.

Luscious Lipstick

The general principle is that either your eyes or your mouth carry the day – never both. Putting on a slick of lipstick, even if the rest of your make-up is very low-key, can bring some much-needed colour to the face and make it look 'dressed' rather than 'naked'.

While there is a limitless colour range to choose from, this does not mean that every colour will suit you. Match lipsticks to your skin tone rather than your clothes and plump for shades which seem to flatter your complexion. Choosing a lipstick on the basis of an article in a magazine can be a bit of lottery, but don't let that stop you experimenting with new colours.

Try different formulations to achieve the effect and level of coverage that you want, from a hint of sheer colour to a deep, matt stain. A lot of research has gone into creating lipsticks which give long-lasting cover while conditioning your lips, so there is no excuse for a product which doesn't work. Renewal

It is important to **ring the changes**: when you wear the same tried and tested lipsticks year after year, you can end up looking as though you are stuck in a time warp.

Lipstick is an important tool for the professional woman and an increasingly valuable prop as we age.

microbeads, the latest innovation in lipstick technology, guarantee to release colour and moisture at regular intervals throughout the day whenever you press your lips together.

There is a knack to applying lipstick which is worth acquiring if you're interested in a professional finish and maximum staying power. These are the basic principles:

- Look after your lips and keep them moist. Even the most sophisticated lipstick formulation cannot make out-of-condition lips look sleek and luscious.

- Outline your lips with a lip pencil to give them a clearly defined edge and stop the colour 'bleeding'. If you cannot match the pencil to your lipstick, use a colourless or natural pencil. Coloured pencils can also be used to fill in your lips for a clean, matt finish.

- A specially designed lip brush will help you to apply colour with precision and make it stick. Blot each layer with a single-ply tissue and build up colour until you are happy with the result. Brush a sprinkling of loose powder over the tissue to 'fix'.

■ To make thin lips look fuller, wear pale colours and add a dab of gloss to the middle of the lips (this makes all lips appear more voluptuous). If your lips are fuller than you'd like, stick to deeper tones and avoid screamingly bright colours and too much shine.

TEETH

The importance of oral hygiene cannot be overemphasized. Unless you protect your teeth and gums with regular and effective brushing and flossing, you are inviting decay and gum disease. Eventually this may mean the loss of teeth and the erosion of underlying tissue and bone.

The purpose of cleaning is to remove the destructive plaque that settles on the surface of teeth and in the spaces between them, also invading the margins between teeth and gums. It is vital that you get rid of this plaque because, if it is allowed to stay on your teeth for more than 24 hours, it produces acids which dissolve the enamel and attack the gums and eventually hardens to form tartar – detectable as dirty yellow lines that appear on teeth near the gum margin. Plaque is also an underlying cause of bad breath and stained teeth as it provides an adhesive surface for potential 'dyes' to cling to.

Gargle every day with a few mouthfuls of warm **salt** water to keep germs and infections at bay (a generous pinch of salt to half a glass of water). You can also invigorate your gums with a salt rub, which will leave your mouth feeling thoroughly refreshed. Keep a supply of finely ground sea salt in a jar on your bathroom shelf.

The Indian habit of chewing **fennel** and **cardamom** seeds after meals helps to prevent tooth decay, gum disease and associated bad breath. Chomping on a handful of **parsley** is a tried and tested method of removing the smell of garlic or other strong-smelling food on the breath.

Apart from booking in for a dental check-up every six months, there are a number of basic steps you can take to safeguard the health of your teeth and gums:

■ Make sure that you are using a toothpaste which contains fluoride.

■ If you are not doing so already, adopt a brushing technique that enables you to concentrate on the margin between your teeth and gums. This usually means angling your brush up for the upper set of teeth and down for the lower set. Softer bristles do a better job than hard ones, which can wear down the enamel on your teeth. Replace your toothbrush as soon as the bristles begin to splay.

To whiten teeth, use bicarbonate of soda on a damp toothbrush and polish until they gleam. Remember, however, that *white* teeth do not exist – teeth are all variations on a shade of cream.

■ Floss between all your teeth several times a week and brush your teeth at least twice a day.

■ Massage your gums by brushing them with your toothbrush. If they bleed, it is a sure sign that they are unhealthy, in which case you should redouble your efforts.

■ To build and maintain strong teeth, you need an adequate supply of calcium and vitamins C and D.

■ We all know that eating sweets is bad for our teeth. This warning can be extended to include sugary drinks, starchy foods, even dried fruit and unsweetened fruit juices hence the importance of frequent brushing.

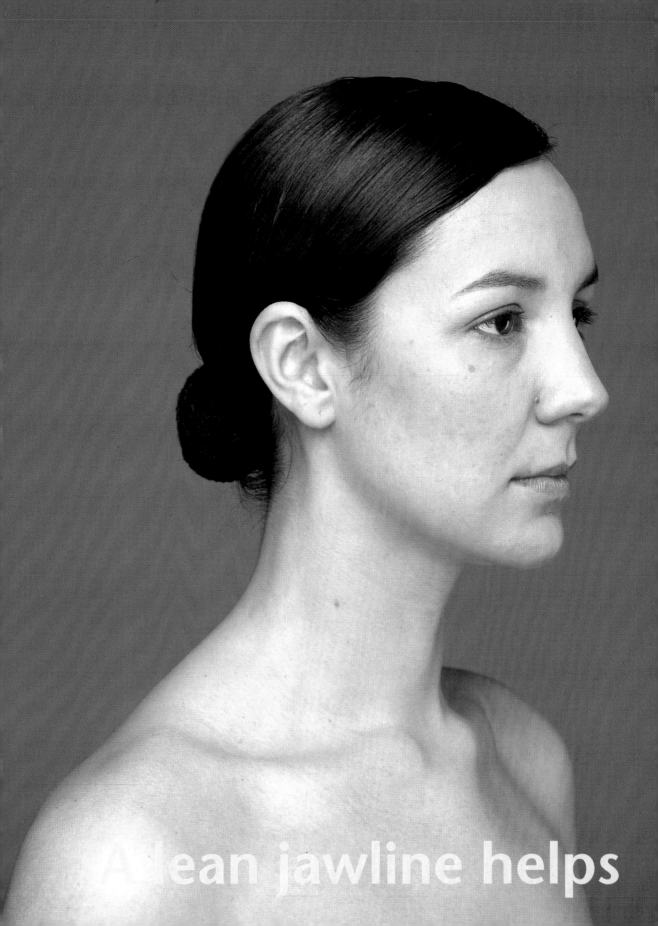

A lean jawline helps

A SMOOTH, slender jawline undoubtedly contributes to an impression of leanness throughout the face, although razor-sharp definition can be harsh and unbecoming. A fleshy jawline, however, blurs the definition of the face and, rightly or wrongly, often signals 'fat'.

By massaging along your jawline, you can prevent stagnation occurring and release a lot of the tension held in this part of the face, which can otherwise lead to headaches and dental problems. Teeth-grinders should make it a regular habit, particularly before bedtime.

The blood supply to the jawline, conveying oxygen and nutrients, is transported from the heart via an upward branch of the aorta, which then subdivides into smaller blood vessels (*see* illustration on page 88). Unlike the branch serving the lower half of our body, the heart has to pump blood up to the jawline and beyond, against the force of gravity. What is more, the main artery supplying blood to our head sub-divides at the jawline, creating a natural stagnation point. It is here, where blood tends to pool, that fat and toxins are also liable to accumulate.

Repeat the following exercise daily to help keep your jawline in trim:

- Rest one elbow on a firm surface and cup your chin in the palm of your hand. Push your chin into the palm, which should resist the pressure.

- Hold for a slow count of five. Repeat five times.

The most common problems with the jawline and chin include:

DOUBLE CHIN

Our jawline is padded out with wider and thicker muscles than our cheeks (*see* illustration on page 170), with a considerable capacity for expansion – hence the problem of double chins. Generally a double chin is a sign of weight gain, although the jawline can also become inflated with fluid and toxins due to sluggish lymphatic circulation.

to *define* your face

You can give yourself a 'false' double chin (and a lot of neck and upper back pain) simply by the way you hold your head. If you retract your chin, it is very easy to create a fold of flesh beneath it, whether you are carrying any extra weight or not. Equally, however, do not over-compensate by jutting out your jaw, as that will impose other, different, strains on the muscles and bones in your neck. The correct position of the head is to have it evenly balanced on top of the neck column (*see* photograph on page 86).

What to Do

- Watch your food intake and cut out 'empty' calories wherever you can.

- Keep up your water consumption, as this will help to sluice out trapped toxins.

Exercise

Limber up your jawline using the following 'pinch and drain' routine.

- Position your thumbs beneath your chin, your three middle fingers of both hands on top, and pinch. Resume your position, press firmly and glide your fingers a little way along your jawline.

- Pinch again and repeat the procedure until you reach the corners of your jawbone. Apply sustained pressure here for a few seconds and just beneath your earlobes.

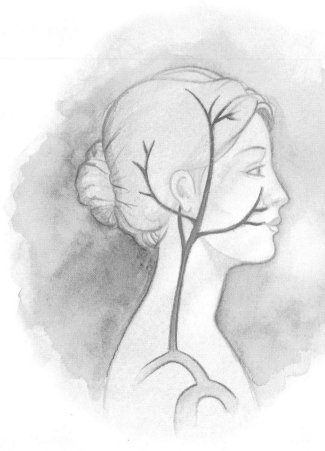

The main arteries leading to the face and scalp.

Get into the habit of doing this at odd times of the day and you should see a dramatic improvement within three months. Once the problem is under control, maintain the effect by repeating the routine as part of your weekly Home Therapy (*see* pages 5–19).

LOOSE SKIN

When tissue is stretched over bone, as it is on our jawline, its elasticity slowly diminishes. The problem of loose skin usually occurs when the jawline has been allowed to become heavy. It is compounded by crash dieting which, typically, results in a rapid loss of weight and flesh, leaving a layer of slack skin which has not been able to contract. Loose skin is also a problem which affects women in middle age battling against the dual effect of increasing body fat and sagging skin.

What to Do

■ Gently stimulate the area using the palms of your hands in a sweeping action, and nourish the skin with almond oil. Repeat night and morning.

> Regular exfoliation with the All-purpose Oatmeal Scrub (*see* page 36) will encourage the regeneration process. Allow three to six months for improvement.

PIGMENTATION

The skin on your chin and along your jawline is particularly exposed due to the prominence of the bone beneath. Potentially harmful ultraviolet rays and damage caused by other 'traumas', such as incompetent electrolysis or mismanaged spots, cause cells lower down in the epidermis to release protective melanin pigments, which leave small marks or larger areas of discoloration on the surface of the skin.

What to Do

The aim is to disperse and encourage even distribution of pigments while avoiding any irritation to your skin:

■ Apply a mild cleansing lotion or almond oil to the area and massage gently using the balls of the first two fingers, paying particular attention to the indentation just above your chin.

■ If you have sensitive skin, use paraffin-based products or almond oil to moisturize. Wear a sunscreen (SPF 15) all year round and switch to a total sun block in the hot summer months.

■ Exfoliate regularly with the Gentle Facial Exfoliator (*see* page 36).

CONGESTED AND SPOTTY SKIN

Sluggish circulation and inefficient lymphatic drainage cause waste to collect in our jawline and pollute surrounding tissue. Hormonal fluctuations also disturb the activities of our sebaceous glands, resulting in overactivity and blockages, leading to blackheads, open pores and spots. This explains why we sometimes get pimples on our chin just before a period.

What to Do

■ Pinch and drain the jawline in the direction of your earlobe, where there is a lymph gland waiting to filter out toxins (*see* above). This routine needs to be carried out two or three times a day until the problem is under control, then once a week to keep the skin clear.

■ Gently massage your chin to disperse any congestion.

■ Avoid touching and picking spots because of the risk of scarring and pigmentation marks.

■ Steer clear of fatty and fried foods and increase your consumption of fresh fruit, vegetables and wholegrains.

■ Aim to drink eight to ten glasses of water daily.

Skincare

The jawline is apt to be overlooked in the cleansing of your face and neck and the chin rarely gets the attention it requires.

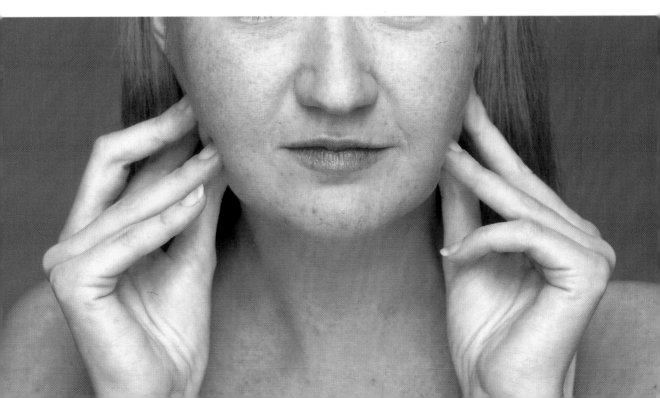

■ Using a mildly medicated soap or a soap-free facial wash, clean the affected area at least twice a day and rinse well.

■ Apply a camphor-based spot treatment as needed.

■ Moisturize with an oil-free formulation.

■ Exfoliate the area once a week using the All-purpose Oatmeal Scrub (*see* page 36).

■ Apply the Healing Mask (*see* page 36).

EXCESS HAIR

Hormonal imbalances during adolescence and after the menopause can cause the normally inconspicuous hairs on our chin and jawline to coarsen and darken. This problem, which often runs in families, can also arise from premature use of the contraceptive pill or be a side-effect of steroid-based medications.

What to Do

I cannot stress enough how important it is to leave facial hair well alone while it is still in its fine, downy state. Once the hairs become bristly and pigmented, however, professional treatment is the safest course of action.

■ I strongly recommend the American TE (Transdermal Electrolysis) system.

Alternatively, hair scanning is another gentle, non-invasive option which, because it is pain-free, is suitable for the treatment of larger areas (*see* page 70 for a description of both methods).

■ Cleanse with a pH-balanced soap or soap-free facial wash and protect with a light water-based moisturizer.

MAKE-UP

■ If you were ever in any doubt about which area of skin to match foundation to, notice the 'tide mark' at the jawline when the shade is mismatched. The skin tone of the neck is approximately the same as that on the inside of the forearms, so test foundation there. If you need to go a little darker for camouflaging purposes, apply colour under the jawline and onto the neck and ears as well.

■ Correct the hollow of the chin, if it is very prominent, using a concealer stick dotted on top of your regular foundation.

■ To minimize a heavy jaw, try sweeping a little darker powder (faceshaper) along the jawline – make sure that you blend it in well. Double chins can also be disguised by brushing darker powder over the fleshy parts.

THE NECK

T HE neck is one of the most naturally graceful – and hard-working – parts of the body. A supple neck makes for a youthful and vivacious appearance. Indeed, the lively head movements of a young person are in many ways a perfect definition of natural beauty.

The underlying muscles play a vital part in preserving the appearance of the skin on our neck which, short on both padding and natural moisture, is often one of the first areas to show signs of ageing. The muscles of our neck are also the repositories for a lot of tension which can undermine the health of the neck tissue. Regular massage and gentle exercise will help to rid the muscles of any toxic build-up while improving their tone. It will also help to keep the joints supple and dispel stores of tension.

Do not wait until you see tell-tale rings and crêpiness appearing on your neck before learning the benefits of protecting this fragile skin from dehydration and environmental damage.

WHAT TO DO

■ Give your neck a weekly massage following the directions in Home Therapy (*see* pages 5–19).

■ To release and realign your neck and shoulders, imagine that your head is being pulled upwards by a piece of string attached to the crown.

■ If you use a VDU (Visual Display Unit), raise the height of it, so that your neck is not permanently inclined as you look at it. Also make a point of holding reading material up before your eyes rather than bending your neck to read it on a flat surface.

■ Sleeping habits can compound posture-related problems. Reduce your pillow height if you feel any strain in your neck. The purpose of a pillow is to fill the gap between your ear and your shoulder while keeping your head at a right angle to your neck.

■ Stimulate the following acupressure point to relieve tension and improve mobility in the neck and shoulders: Gall Bladder 20 (*see* page 35).

A supple neck helps to

enhance *ageless* beauty

SKINCARE & MAKE-UP

■ Your neck needs to be cleansed night and morning in the same way as your face, starting at the collarbones and working up to the jawline.

■ Apply a rich moisturizing cream at night and a moisturizer combined with sunscreen during the day. Do not forget to include the sides of your neck and the area around the collarbones.

■ Exfoliate your neck once a week using the All-purpose Oatmeal Scrub (*see* page 36).

■ If using a foundation darker than your natural skin tone for camouflage purposes, apply to your neck and ears as well.

Common problems affecting the neck include:

CREPEY NECK

This is when the thin skin on the neck – no longer held taut – is covered by a network of fine lines. There is often a build-up of dead cells on the surface as well. The problem is usually a symptom of ageing or prematurely aged skin due to lost muscle tone, although the skin can deteriorate in this way after a long period of ill health. It also tends to be more acute with fair skin and most noticeable on long necks.

What to Do

■ Exfoliate your skin daily with the All-purpose Oatmeal Scrub (*see* page 36) for an initial period of three weeks, then reducing to once a week.

■ Apply almond oil as a nourishing moisturizer.

Exercise
The following exercises, performed daily, will strengthen and firm neck muscles. Sit well-supported in an upright chair:

■ Keeping your chin level, turn your head to one side so that the chin is over your shoulder. Incline the head backwards in a 'come hither' movement (*see* below). Repeat on the other side. Repeat the sequence five times.

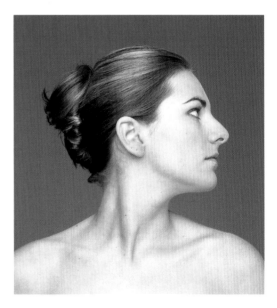

■ Hold your head in a central position, then lean it as far over as you can towards one shoulder and hold for a count of 10 (*see* below). Your neck may feel rather stiff to begin with. Repeat on the other side, making sure that your shoulders remain still and relaxed throughout. Do five repetitions.

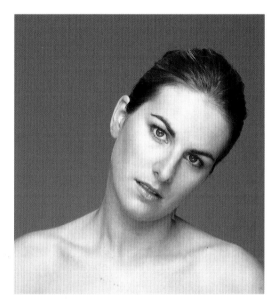

GOOSEPIMPLY NECK

This occurs when the small bundles of muscle alongside the hair follicles, which cause goosepimples, are permanently irritated and, therefore, contracted due to some internal stimulus. Increased toxicity in the area as a result of a surge in hormones, particularly the chemicals released by stress, is most commonly to blame.

What to Do

■ While in this state, the capacity of the follicles to absorb moisture will be greatly reduced, so restrict yourself to a very light moisturizer to soften the skin.

■ Exfoliate as above. Repeat daily for two to three months. The neck tissue will become smooth again as toxins are carried away by brisker lymphatic circulation.

■ Practise the following neck exercise several times a day: clench your jaws, stretch your mouth sideways and hold for a count of 10.

■ Drink eight to ten glasses of water daily.

IRREGULAR PIGMENTATION

This problem occurs on the neck for all the usual reasons including sun damage and a high level of toxicity in the body. Also, when our head carriage is poor and we allow our neck to sink into our bodies, we create deep creases in our neck which end up as distinct rings of lighter skin because of the uneven distribution of melanin pigment.

What to Do

■ Always hold yourself as tall and straight as you can and extend your neck to its maximum length.

- Apply almond oil sparingly to your neck and massage in an upwards direction using a gentle 'palming' action (*see* page 7).

- To disperse melanin build-up, exfoliate your neck once a week with the All-purpose Oatmeal Scrub (*see* page 36), using the minimum finger pressure.

EXCESS HAIR

Profuse hair growth following the male pattern usually occurs when there is a surfeit of male hormones in the body, in which case hairs on our neck (generally around the Adam's apple) often accompany hairs on the chin. However, irritation to the skin caused by woollen scarves and high-necked sweaters, particularly if there is an allergy to wool, can result in odd hairs sprouting on our neck. Steroid medicines and creams may equally be at the root of the problem.

What to Do

- Remember that the shallow neck tissue is easily scarred by misguided attempts to remove hair, so seek professional help if you want a permanent solution to the problem (*see* page 70).

- The treatment for downy hairs is to rub gently with a towel from an early age or bleach naturally with fresh lemon juice (*see* page 55).

FATTY NECK

This is usually associated with hormonal or thyroid problems (which may be accompanied by a bulging Adam's apple) and is much more common with shorter necks. Excess weight may also be the cause.

What to Do

- If it is caused by a weight increase, a stimulating massage every evening, in addition to the exercises described above (*see* page 94), will help to disperse the fat.

Chronic tension in the muscles at the base of the neck and across the shoulders needs urgent and regular attention. Massage relieves and revives the area by restoring the blood supply and flushing out the toxins responsible for the discomfort. Rub lightly up and down each shoulder using the palm of the opposite hand until you feel the muscles beginning to unclench. Continue for up to five minutes. You can do this treatment virtually anywhere at any time.

- Apply a light film of almond oil all over your neck and, using all four fingers, 'pinch' the front, sides and back for a few minutes. Continue daily for a period of three months, increasing or decreasing frequency according to the level of fat build-up.

SHOULDERS

Our natural shoulder line is often distorted by the impact of our emotions on our physical bearing, as well as by physical wear and tear. We carry more tension in our shoulders than in any other part of the body. Apart from causing intense discomfort, this can create hard, prominent muscles that add unnecessary bulk to our appearance.

Use a moisturizer with a built-in sunscreen on your neck all year round and a high factor (SPF 15+) in the summer. Do not overlook the sides of your neck.

When we hunch our shoulders in response to feelings of anxiety, we contract the large trapezius muscle. Shoulders habitually rounded in a defensive stance cause the deltoid muscles to become rigid and the pectorals to become permanently shortened (*see* muscle illustration on page 173). However, ramming the shoulders back in response to requests to 'straighten up' our posture is equally unhealthy and unnatural. The aim is to persuade your shoulders to sink down and back, so that your arms hang naturally by your sides.

Carrying heavy and unevenly distributed loads also creates problems and can result in one shoulder sitting permanently higher than the other.

What to Do

- Our shoulders are capable of a huge range of movement which we need to preserve. Shrugging your shoulders (out of choice, rather than despair) is a good way of maintaining mobility. Whenever I have a spare moment, I shrug alternate shoulders in time to the music I am listening to. Such rhythmical movements really help the muscles to relax.

- Weekly Home Therapy (*see* pages 5–19) will help to keep the problem under control.

- Refer to page 119 for guidelines on correct posture.

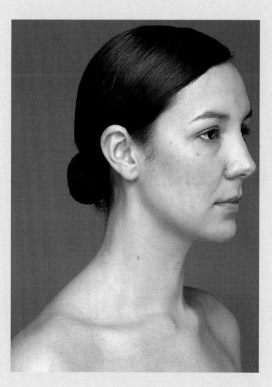

There is someth*i*ng *lovely*

UPPER ARMS

THERE is something particularly attractive about a lean, well-toned upper arm. It gives the impression of a healthy, active body. By contrast, flabby, flaccid arms suggests sluggishness and inertia. Since the muscles of the upper arms move the forearms and bear most of the load when you are lifting an object, there are plenty of opportunities to put these muscles to work, without having to book in at the local gym.

COMMON PROBLEMS

■ Goosepimply skin – irritated sebaceous glands cause permanent erection of the muscles on either side of the follicles. The most common reason for this is a build-up of toxins due to inefficient circulation.

■ Flabby upper arms – a result of a build-up of fluid and toxins around fatty deposits, aggravated by sluggish circulation.

■ Loose skin – caused by rapid loss of muscle tone and underlying fat as a result of crash dieting.

■ Slack muscle tone – due to lack of exercise or failure to maintain a muscle once it has been toned.

■ Irregular pigmentation – generally caused by overexposure to sun or hormonal imbalance.

■ Dry, flaky skin – caused by sun damage or hormonal imbalance within the body due to a thyroid condition. Extreme dryness may also be linked to eczema or psoriasis.

WHAT TO DO

■ A regular Dead Sea salt bath (*see* page 22) will provide instant relief and on-going therapy for troublesome joints, over-worked muscles or fluid retention in the arms, as well as restoring skin to a peachy softness. The resulting improved blood supply will ensure that the skin tone is even, rather than patchy or ghostly white.

■ All of the above conditions require daily exfoliation to slough off dead skin cells and activate peripheral nerve endings. Use the All-purpose Oatmeal Scrub

about a lean upper arm

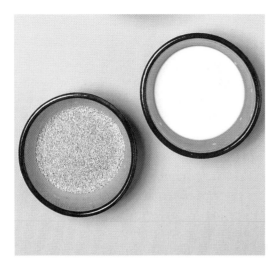

FOREARMS

We use the muscles of our forearms when we grasp objects – everything from a tennis racquet to a cup of tea. Since these muscles are often required to carry heavy loads, tension and strain can be a problem. Try to relax them regularly with gentle massage – it is important.

COMMON PROBLEMS

■ Weak and tired muscles – due to poor circulation or overuse.

■ Prematurely aged skin – a result of sun damage or the side effects of long-term medication.

■ Pigmentation marks – a reaction to sun damage or hormonal imbalance.

■ Dry skin – caused by poor circulation and neglect.

■ Hairy arms – dark hairs make normal growth appear more conspicuous. Superabundant growth and coarse hairs indicate a hormonal imbalance.

What to Do

■ Using upward strokes, rub olive or almond oil into the skin of your forearm after your bath or before you go to bed. Continue for two to three

(*see* page 36) or one of the numerous exfoliating preparations available on the market. This will get the skin to function properly and assist the work carried out beneath the surface by the lymphatic, circulatory and nervous systems.

■ Give the upper arm a regular massage with almond or olive oil (*see* page 15).

The following gentle exercise is designed to build long, lean biceps and triceps:

■ Raise your arms in line with your shoulder, with your palms facing down.

■ Make a fist, squeeze and hold for a count of ten.

■ Release and repeat five times.

minutes. This will help dry skin and soothe weak and tired muscles.

■ For uneven pigmentation, use a sun block or cover up when in the very hot sun. Always wear a sunscreen in direct sunlight to guard against further markings.

■ Stimulate the following acupressure point to improve the mobility of the forearm: Large Intestine 11 (*see* page 29).

■ If hairy arms are a problem, waxing is very effective for clearing the area and reducing growth.

HANDS

Graceful, silky hands and beautiful nails are much-prized, physical attributes. Supple hands and trim, healthy nails speak volumes about our state of health and personal grooming. Neglected hands, however, rather let the side down. And they don't just create a poor impression – they can belie our age.

Our hands are in the front line and bear the brunt of extreme weather conditions and, even worse, cannot escape constant contact with water and detergents. The strength of our nails is also undermined by the damaging effects of water, which causes the substance which bonds the nail cells to dissolve and our nails to flake.

Even if we remember to arm ourselves with rubber gloves when washing up, our hands still remain vulnerable. The skin on our hands, especially on our fingertips, is one of the most sensitive areas in the body. Over time, repeated exposure to water and extreme weather conditions without adequate protection can result in dehydration and permanent discoloration of the skin, in other words, prematurely aged hands.

The only effective way to preserve our hands and screen them from external damage is by creating a barrier between them and the outside world. So, don't stint on the hand cream – even if you think your hands are still in their prime. If, however, you're convinced that they're over the hill, every bit of extra protection will contribute to their rehabilitation – which can be surprisingly swift.

I believe very strongly in the value of using our hands therapeutically. It is important for everybody to know their skin and its changing textures. Unless you have felt the velvety texture of thriving skin, you will not really know when it is below par. To be able to do this, you need healthy hands.

Good circulation to the hands is also vital to keep joints mobile and build strong, smooth nails. Be aware too that if you allow dead skin cells to build up, joints to stiffen and hands to become sore and lifeless, they will not work as well for you.

101

COMMON PROBLEMS

- Dry, flaky skin – see earlier for causes. If the problem is not rectified the skin may also become slack.

- Pigmentation – caused by sun damage, hormonal imbalance, ill health or ageing, for example.

- Hairy knuckles and backs of hands – due to hormonal imbalance, side effects of androgen or steroid drugs, heredity. More common from the late forties onwards.

- Icy hands with distorted flesh tone – a combination of poor circulation and fine skin allows bluish colour of blood to show through.

- Stiff hands – caused by tension due to overuse, weakness arising from injury, underuse or arthritic joints.

- Puffy hands – a symptom of fluid retention in the tissues due to poor circulation.

What to Do

- Always wear gloves for household tasks that involve immersing your hands in water, for gardening and in cold weather.

- Use a heavy barrier cream to help protect the skin from dehydration. Keep a supply by every sink at home. Apply a slick whenever your hands have come into contact with water and always last thing at night. Glycerine-based hand creams are non-greasy and help to rehydrate the skin (glycerine is a humectant – that is, it attracts moisture from the air.)

- In the summer, or if you spend a lot of time outside, add a layer of sunscreen to your hands, or look for a hand cream with a built-in SPF. With pigmentation problems, it is advisable to wear a high-factor sunscreen all year round.

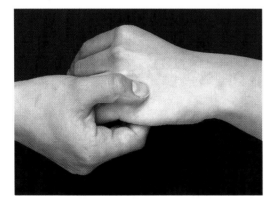

Every time you use handcream give your hands a **mini-therapy**:

Rub cream into your knuckles and finger joints using small circular movements, followed by a pulling motion to ease the joints.

Now use your thumbs to massage the backs of the hands upwards in the direction of the wrist to clear any congestion (*see* left).

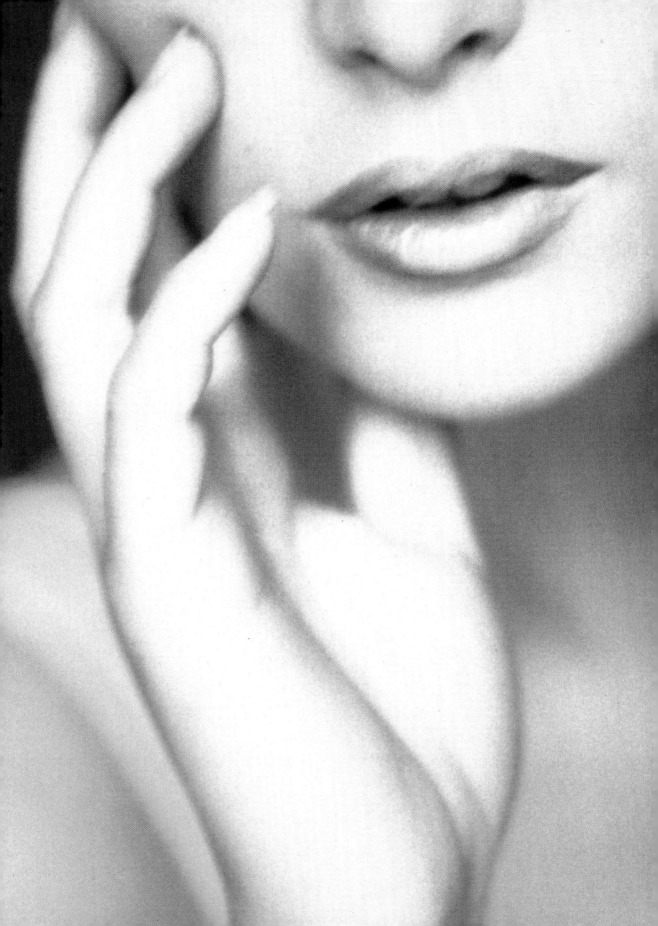

Soak your hands in salt water for 15–20 minutes every day for a two week period to relieve stiff, aching hands and reduce any swelling or puffiness. The most effortless way to do this while in the bath (*see* page 22). Rinse with fresh water and push back the cuticles with a damp flannel.

■ Exfoliate your hands daily for three weeks using a mineral peel or the All-purpose Oatmeal Scrub (*see* page 36). Watch your hands undergo a transformation as successive layers of dried out, dead skin cells are stripped away to reveal fresh new ones beneath. Regular exfoliation will also reduce the intensity of pigmentation marks and normalize the circulation, encouraging a more even distribution of pigments. Repeat weekly to maintain.

■ Unsightly hairs on knuckles or backs of hands can either be removed permanently by electrolysis or waxed (which will gradually weaken growth).

NAILS

Even if long, painted talons are not our heart's desire, possessing bitten, broken or stunted nails can make us extremely self-conscious about our hands. Do not despair, however, the outlook is far from bleak.

Hair and nails (which are, in effect, layers of modified skin cells) share many characteristics and flourish on a similar regime. Both benefit from a well-balanced diet – packed with vitamins and minerals and including an adequate supply of proteins – and suffer when our health is poor. As we age, and the chemical balance of our bodies changes, our nails become thicker and more brittle. They also become less able to retain moisture. The good habits which help to preserve your hands will also protect your nails.

The cuticle – the thin membrane that grows between the nail and the skin of the nail fold – is designed to stop infection, dirt and debris invading the nail bed and should be treated with great care. As long as cuticles are well-nourished and the skin is supple, they should not require any special attention. However, if they start to overhang the nail or become dehydrated, ease them back gently using a flannel when they are nicely softened after a soak in the bath. Alternatively, use a cotton wool bud after applying cream or oil. Resist the temptation to cut cuticles.

COMMON PROBLEMS

■ Soft nails – when nail cells are over-watered and underfed due to inefficient circulation. Flimsy nails offer the nail bed less protection and are more prone to damage.

- Brittle nails – generally caused by a dehydrated nail bed or a shortage of calcium or EFAs (essential fatty acids) in the diet, although brittle nails are sometimes linked to an immune-related condition.

- Dehydrated, flaky and splitting nails – caused by neglect, poor circulation and a shortage of vitamins and/or proteins in the diet. Chlorinated water and some nail varnish removers also have a drying effect on nails.

- Ridges in nails – due to injury, vitamin deficiency or simply ageing. Very pronounced cases may be caused by a fungal infection.

- White spots – often signify damage or overenthusiastic manicuring, although they may indicate a zinc deficiency.

- Rough nails – the surface of the nails becomes grainy when dead cells are allowed to accumulate.

- Discoloration or staining from nicotine, for example – this can be a problem if the nail is dehydrated, as the porous layers of cells that make up the nail soak up the colour more easily. If nails turn yellow due to natural causes, it is a indication of poor health.

What to Do

Massage hand cream into your nails, cuticles and the tops of your fingers below the free edges of your nails using small thumb rotations.

Apply a nourishing cream or oil every night before you go to bed. Almond oil is a particularly good nail food and will soak easily into your hands if applied just after a bath.

- Unless your nails are in mint condition, wear them no longer than the tips of your fingers, to keep them manageable. Squareish ends and straight sides look modern and practical.

Keep your nails clean. Whatever nail problems you are grappling with, this is one area you have complete control over. There is no substitute for a daily scrub with a good nail brush.

- File nails regularly (preferably with a large 'professional' emery board), using the rough side to shorten and the smooth side to shape. Work upwards in one direction, rather than 'sawing' back and forth, as friction weakens the layers of the nails, causing them to split. If you want to shorten nails dramatically, clip across the top, then file the sides to desired shape.

■ Nails also benefit from weekly exfoliation with the same preparation you use on your hands, to smooth the surface and encourage regeneration of new cells. Pay particular attention to the base of the nail, around the cuticle, where dead cells often accumulate.

All the problems listed earlier will benefit from the following routine. The frictional heat which is generated improves the flow of blood to the nail bed, assuring the delivery of nutrients and oxygen essential for strong, healthy nail growth:

■ Bend the fingers of both hands in towards the palms and press the nails together. Keeping your hands relaxed, rub the two sets of fingernails against one another for one minute – your thumbs will be a bit hit and miss.

■ Repeat this process regularly. Even if poor nail condition is a result of an underlying medical condition, more efficient circulation can assist the nourishing and repairing process.

■ If you have a tendency to flaky, chipped, dehydrated or thickened nails, file the free edges of the nails daily and apply a nail strengthener every night to hold the cell layers together. If your nails are at all brittle, avoid any formulation containing formaldehyde.

■ Apply a base coat to fill in any irregularities on the surface of the nails. It will also provide a protective layer and prevent staining. Wipe off any drops that spill onto cuticles.

■ Filling in the underside of the nail with a white nail pencil can make unpainted nails look prettier.

Use nail varnish to shield the nails while they are on the mend. You may notice some improvement after as little as a week if your nails have been neglected, but be patient. It will probably take six months to rectify long-standing problems. Once your nails have been restored, maintain them weekly using the Home Spa and Home Therapy routines.

When they are back in peak condition, allow nails to go bare for a few days every month so that they can 'breathe'.

Painting Nails

- Remove all traces of grease with soap and water before painting.

- Make sure that the brush is not over-loaded and that there is no varnish on the stem. Apply varnish using three strokes – side, middle, side – starting with the little finger and working towards the thumb.

- Beware of using dark colours, as any irregularities will be highlighted if the varnish is not well-applied. Light, metallic colours are practical because pits and grooves are less conspicuous. They also look less shabby when the varnish chips.

- Remove varnish with acetone-free remover, which is much kinder to nails.

BUST & MIDRIFF

THE BUST

A GREAT deal of anxiety surrounds the whole issue of breast size and shape, and myths abound about how it is possible to make the bust more voluptuous. Our breasts consist of fat and fibrous connective tissue arranged around milk-producing ducts. The proportion of fat cells – which is what makes breast size vary – is dictated by hereditary factors, weight and the natural shape of our body and can only be increased by a good diet.

> Improving your posture is the first easy step towards creating a beautiful bustline, as good posture lifts the ribcage naturally upwards and outwards and makes the breasts sit a little prouder on the chest. Correct posture is also essential to stop heavy breasts from exerting a strain on the upper back and shoulders.

There is no muscular tissue within our breasts to hold them up; they are supported by the pectoral muscles which lie between the breasts and the ribcage (*see* page 96). Well-toned pectorals provide sturdier underpinnings for an ample bust, and will also bolster a small bust.

Our breasts are subject to fluctuations in volume and weight dictated by hormonal changes in the body. In the latter half of the menstrual cycle, fluid seeps into the fatty tissue causing the breasts to become fuller and heavier – and often a little tender. Breasts enlarge considerably during pregnancy, when they are being prepared to produce milk, and expand still further when the milk arrives. It is advisable to keep the skin on the breasts as supple as possible to avoid the appearance of stretch marks.

COMMON PROBLEMS

■ Spotty chest – triggered by hormonal fluctuations during puberty, the menopause and within the menstrual cycle itself. Picking and squeezing spots can result in the formation of unsightly keloid scars.

■ Sagging breasts – very heavy or inadequately supported breasts pull on the ligaments causing them to stretch. Droopy breasts are generally due to

Improve your posture

for a *curvaceous bust*

rapid weight-loss, the loss of fat cells after the menopause or breastfeeding.

- Hairy nipples – it is quite common to have the odd hair growing around the nipple, but hormonal changes triggered by the contraceptive pill and the menopause may increase the growth.

- Inverted nipples – nipples fail to pop out because they are stuck to the underlying structure of the breast.

- Stretch marks – a problem of lost elasticity in the skin, usually due to a surge of adrenal hormones. Stretch marks commonly appear in adolescence and during pregnancy, when the bust expands significantly.

Hydrotherapy (treatment using hot and cold water) can restore tone to breasts by bringing more blood to the surface and encouraging activity in the tissue. Apply an ice-cold compress – a suitably sized towel or piece of cloth soaked in icy water and squeezed out – to droopy or diminutive breasts, or expose them to a cold water spray, for just under a minute. Repeat several times, twice a day. Over-full breasts will benefit from a couple of long, hot applications (up to five minutes), sandwiched in between short cold ones. Repeat twice a day for three weeks and then twice weekly until you are happier with them.

What to Do

- Eat a balanced diet with plenty of fresh fruit, vegetables and whole-grains and include a variety of the following proteins: fish, poultry, lean meat, eggs, nuts and pulses. Eat your daily quota of favourable fats (*see* page 161).

- A vitamin E supplement can help to relieve breast tenderness and may reduce your susceptibility to stretch marks during vulnerable periods. Rubbing the contents of a vitamin E capsule into the skin may help to keep stretch marks at bay.

■ Get your bra size checked from time to time, particularly after a substantial increase or decrease in weight.

■ If the downy hairs around the nipple start to become wiry and strong (which can happen if you pluck them), it is advisable to have them removed professionally by electrolysis (*see* page 79).

■ To help release inverted nipples, place one thumb above and one below the nipple and gently pull on it six times. Repeat with your thumbs on the other side. Do this several times a day.

SKINCARE

■ The fine skin which covers your breasts needs to be regularly moisturized. Using the palms of your hands (or your fingers if you have small breasts), apply almond oil or body lotion, moving upwards around the breasts, lifting each one gently so that you can massage the underside, and sweeping up into your armpits. This helps to clear toxins from the breast tissue while assisting the firming process. When in the sun, protect the area with a high factor sunscreen.

■ Exfoliate the bust, excluding the nipples, once a week with the All-purpose Oatmeal Scrub (*see* page 36). Increase

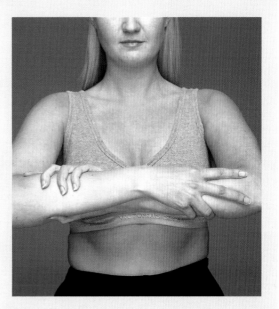

Exercise

Do the following exercise night and morning. Once you feel your bust start to firm up, reduce to three or four times a week:

■ Stretch your arms out in front of you, bend them at the elbow and grasp each forearm firmly below the elbow with the opposite hand (*see* above).

■ Breathe in slowly through your nose and, as you breathe out, tighten your grip and hold for a count of five, increasing to ten. Repeat ten times.

This will strengthen the underlying pectorals as well as guarding against 'back tyres'. If you can fit swimming into your routine, the fittingly named breaststroke is a great bust-enhancer.

111

to three times a week if the skin is unhealthy. Massage using firm, circular movements, as this will enliven the circulation, dislodge dry, dead skin cells and disperse stagnant pigments.

■ Apply a Healing Mask (*see* page 36) to spots as needed and leave for up to 30 minutes before rinsing off.

MIDRIFF

We are all very conscious of our tummies and fluctuating girths, and may well envy the washboard stomachs of the adolescent models we see in the pages of glossy magazines. In fact, there is something very feminine about a slightly rounded tummy, and most of us feel that a less angular silhouette is a fair trade-off for the pleasures brought by children and a life lived to the full. What we do need to guard against, however, is the progressive loss of muscle tone in the abdominal area, which has implications for our health as well as our figures.

The waist curve marks the narrowest point in the middle of our trunk where our ribcage ends and our hips begin. Waists acquire definition during adolescence, when the female body assumes its womanly contours, and gradually thicken with the passing of the years. A trim waist is something to be proud of and to hang on to, for a whole

host of reasons. The much-bemoaned inclination of the pear-shaped figure to carry extra weight on the hips and thighs does have benefits for our health, while the tendency of the apple-shaped figure to expand around the middle, laying down stores of fat around the vital organs, has come to be associated with an increased risk of heart disease, diabetes and both breast and endometrial cancer.

Clearly, in order to preserve your waistline, you need to avoid any unnecessary weight gain, although abdominal distension can occur as a result of a clogged digestive system or food intolerance. Wheat, dairy products and yeast are common culprits, so try cutting these out (*see* page 157). That said, a few extra pounds should not get in the way of a firm and shapely midriff, provided that your posture is well-aligned and the underlying muscles are in reasonable shape. After childbirth, the natural elasticity of the stomach muscles helps them to contract, especially if they are activated fairly soon afterwards. Until the skin and underlying muscles return to their pre-pregnancy state – and this takes longer with successive pregnancies – the stomach is likely to have a loose and slightly baggy appearance.

There are four layers of muscles running vertically, diagonally and horizontally beneath the skin of the abdomen which, when firm, act as a natural corset (*see* page 112). A large number of important organs – the stomach, liver, spleen, kidneys, intestines, uterus and ovaries – lie in the abdominal cavity beneath. When our abdominal muscles are weak, these internal organs are not properly protected and supported, which can impair their function and contribute indirectly to problems such as constipation and painful periods. Slack stomach muscles also place an extra burden on our lower back.

COMMON PROBLEMS

■ Loose muscle tone – due to poor posture, sedentary habits and lack of exercise. Also occurs post-pregnancy.

■ Over-stretched skin and stretch marks – the problem of lost elasticity, described earlier in this section, often appearing during adolescence and pregnancy when the abdomen expands significantly.

> Regular swimming using a range of strokes will help to streamline abdominal and back muscles.

■ Dry skin – occurs as a result of a build-up of dead cells, dehydration from excessive sunbathing or a shortage of EFAs in the diet. It is also an early warning signal of disharmony within the body.

■ Pigmented skin – overtight clothing around the waist restricts the blood supply and irritates the skin, both

of which cause pigments to settle here.

■ Premenstrual bloating – due to a high level of oestrogen in the blood.

What to Do

■ Activate the flesh on your abdomen using brisk pinching movements. This will improve the tone of the muscles, as well as mobilizing fat cells. Do it after your bath, having first lubricated the skin with body lotion or oil.

> Watch your posture and practise the pelvic tilt described on page 119 until it becomes second nature. Notice how your stomach instantly looks flatter and your silhouette more streamlined. Holding the pelvis in position involves a continuous but gentle contraction of the stomach and buttock muscles, which helps to tighten them up and provide support for your spine (*see* illustration on page 119).

■ Take daily salt baths in the week leading up to menstruation to disperse any fluid build-up. Carry out your own lymphatic drainage by rubbing a face cloth slowly and firmly up your legs from your ankle to your groin.

■ If you have a tendency to pigmentation or dry skin, exfoliate the skin

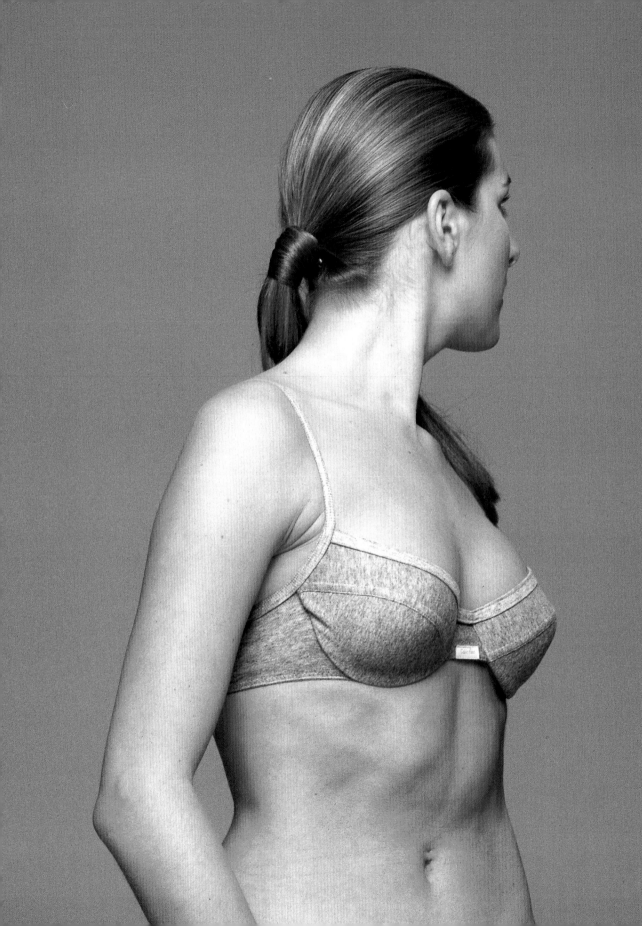

regularly using the All-purpose Oatmeal Scrub (*see* page 36).

■ For stretch marks, increase your intake of vitamin E in food or supplement form during vulnerable periods. This will reduce your susceptibility. You could also pierce a vitamin E capsule, squeeze out its contents and rub into the skin of the abdomen.

If you feel yourself expanding at the waist, take a close look at your diet. Drink plenty of water to flush out the system and eat as much fresh fruit and vegetables as you can. Ensure that there is enough roughage in your diet to keep your digestive tract healthy and prevent constipation. Cut down on cakes, puddings, alcohol and too many fatty and salty processed foods.

Exercise

For your abdominal 'corset' to hold you firmly in place, all four of the superficial abdominal muscles need to be worked. Do the following exercises daily until you see an improvement. Then reduce to three or four times a week to maintain the effect.

■ This is the yoga posture known as *Uddiyana Bandha*. Standing comfortably with your legs apart, bend your body forwards and rest your hands on your thighs. Allow your chin to drop towards your chest and breathe in (*see* below).

Now breathe out and, as you get to the end of the breath, pull your abdominal muscles upwards and backwards towards your chest.

Do this in stages until you have scooped up every last bit of muscle and hold for as long as you can. At the start, you may only be able to manage this exercise once or twice. Aim in the long run for five repetitions.

■ Stand with your hands hanging loosely by your sides and your legs shoulder-width apart. Twist and rotate your trunk at the waist, so that you are looking over your left shoulder. Now twist and look over your right shoulder (*see* left).

Repeat 10 times on each side, edging further round as you loosen up. Breathe slowly and deeply throughout.

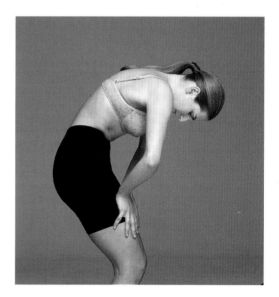

BACK, HIPS & BUTTOCKS

THE BACK

THE back is a strong and beautiful part of the body – a pleasingly smooth expanse and a perfectly designed piece of machinery. We very rarely bare our backs to the world and yet there is something breathtaking about the sight of a firm, blemish-free back revealed in a low-cut dress or skimpy summer top.

The muscles of the back, although you may hardly be aware of them, require conscientious maintenance. Backs may not appear to be a fleshy part of the body and yet 'back tyres' are a relatively common – and avoidable – problem. They develop when the latissimus dorsi muscle has been allowed to become slack and flabby due to inactivity and poor posture.

The biggest favour that you can do for your back – and for your figure – is to become aware of your posture, and learn how to make it work for you rather than against you. Your silhouette is, to a large extent, determined by your posture. When you hold yourself in the right way, you will find that your body creates graceful lines, your movements are fluid and your back is far less susceptible to damage.

COMMON PROBLEMS

■ Back tyres – see above.

■ Lower back problems – a very common complaint capable of causing great pain and a reduction in mobility. We must learn to understand how to help the supporting muscles of our backs through improved circulation and muscle tone, as these can assist the repair and recovery process, as well as preventing back problems from occurring in the first place.

What to Do

■ Always bend your knees and keep your back straight when you reach down to pick something up. Keep any object you lift as close to the body as possible.

■ Regular exercise – and that doesn't have to mean punishing sessions at the gym – is essential to keep your back muscles in condition and ward off back problems. We need to *use* our joints and muscles to keep them healthy. Make it part of your life. You will find swimming, yoga and gentle

Work on your muscles

to *support* your spine

stretching exercises particularly valuable for strengthening the back.

■ Strong stomach muscles take a lot of the strain off our lower back, so do not neglect them (*see* page 115). The powerful buttock muscles also have a vital supporting role to play in relation to our back – another reason to keep them firm and taut.

■ Stretch wholeheartedly and uninhibitedly whenever you get the urge. This action will decompress the spine and trim the midriff. It is also the perfect way to ease your body into action at the beginning of the day and to revive flagging energy levels.

■ Whenever possible wear comfortable shoes which do not throw your spine out of alignment. Alternate high-heeled shoes with flat ones.

■ Sleeping on a firm mattress can ease back pain. If yours is too soft, put a piece of hardboard underneath. Limit yourself to one flattish pillow.

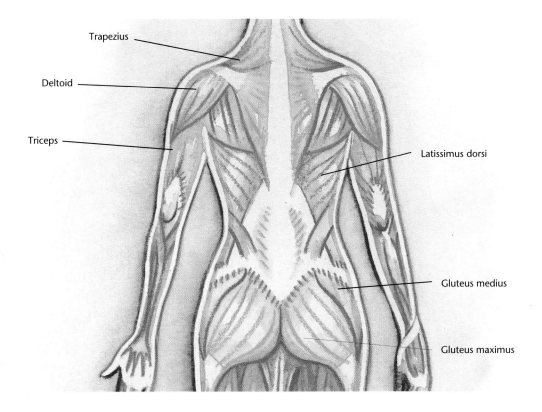

The back and buttock muscles.

Improve your Posture

Work on your standing and sitting posture and be aware of when your back is arched or rounded in a slump. The idea is to preserve the gentle, natural curves in your spine.

Good posture pivots on the correct pelvic tilt because, when the pelvis is balanced, the spine is subject to minimum stress. It is achieved by tucking your bottom under and pulling your tummy in towards your spine (*see* below).

When you are sitting, your upper back should be straight and your lower back angled slightly forwards (*see* overleaf). A small cushion slipped into the small of your back may help to balance your pelvis.

The following technique will help you to shrug off old postural habits.

■ Stand squarely on the outside of your feet and imagine that there are roots descending from your heels deep into the ground. Imagine, too, that there is a tail attached to your tailbone, which pulls down on the end of your spine and encourages it to sink with the force of gravity. At the same time, visualize a piece of string extending upwards from the crown of your head, stretching your spine and making you taller and leaner. This is the 'plumb line' which travels down the spine through the pelvis – the body's centre of gravity – towards the ground.

Once you focus on your spine in this way, you should find that you release your head, arms, neck and shoulders automatically, as you shift the attention away from them.

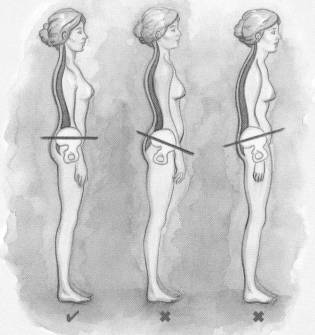

Standing postures showing correct and incorrect pelvic tilt and the alignment of the spine.

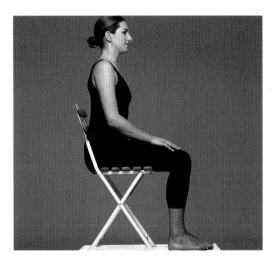

Well-aligned sitting posture.

HIPS

Our hips are a wonderful, womanly feature of our bodies, and yet most of us perceive them as a problem area. The fact is that all women are biologically programmed to store fat around the hips for use in times of need, although some have a greater tendency to stockpile than others. Hips expand twice naturally in a woman's life: first, with the hormonal changes that occur at the onset of puberty, when our hips acquire the padding which gives them their contours; and subsequently, during pregnancy, when the hips widen to accommodate the growing child and open to give birth.

COMMON PROBLEMS

■ Fat build-up – caused by a sedentary lifestyle, hormonal changes, poor diet or overeating. Exacerbated by poor circulation, which allows fat and toxins to settle on the hips.

■ Hip joint problems – possibly due to arthritis, general wear and tear, advancing age, low oestrogen levels post-menopause contributing to osteoporosis or the side effects of medication.

What to Do

■ Massage the flesh daily on the hips using large pinching movements for five minutes on each side. This increases the circulation and helps to break down fat. It will also improve the mobility of the hips by dispersing toxins which undermine the health of joints.

Exercise

It is important to keep the hip area mobile by exercising. Try to take regular, brisk walks and practise the following hip rotations daily:

■ Stand with your feet shoulder-width apart, your bottom tucked in and your shoulders relaxed.

■ Rest your hands on your hips and circle them five times slowly in a clockwise direction, then five times anti-clockwise.

BUTTOCKS

The gluteus muscles in our buttocks (*see* page 118), the most powerful muscles in the body, often carry a huge burden of emotional tension, as well as unwelcome fat and waste. Massage and regular exercise can banish both. It is well worth the effort – a pair of firm, nicely rounded buttocks can really enhance the figure.

COMMON PROBLEMS

- Loose buttocks – due to lack of exercise, sedentary habits, rapid weight-loss and bed rest as a result of illness.

- Cellulite – a circulatory and lifestyle problem. The buttocks attract deposits of fat which become laden with toxins and waste. Exacerbated by poor muscle tone.

- Pigmentation – more common in darker skins, is caused by stagnation in the tissues due to poor circulation, a build-up of dead cells, hormonal imbalance, medication accelerating the production of melanin cells and illness.

What to Do

- Exfoliate your buttocks at bath times using a mildly abrasive mitt, lubricated with a squirt of bath gel. This will remove dead cells and help to even out the skin's pigments. Moisturize well afterwards.

- Massage in your body lotion using small pinching movements. This activates nerve endings in the skin, which enhances muscle tone and aids detoxification.

Exercise

You will be amazed at the toning effect of regular buttock-clenching. Get into the habit of tightening your buttocks, whether standing or sitting, every time you think of it:

- Stand with the pelvis well-balanced and the upper body relaxed. Now really squeeze the buttocks, so that the cheeks are pulled together. This will tighten up muscle tone and help to release stored toxins. Your stomach muscles should benefit too, as they are automatically pulled in at the same time. Make this a way of life – use a dot on your wrist as a cue to remind you.

Walk on your bottom at least three times a week, ten movements forwards, followed by ten backwards, using your arms to help you move. Repeat five times. Apart from working the buttock – and leg – muscles, this also promotes a feeling of general wellbeing and helps to disperse cellulite. Stair-climbing is also good for the buttocks, so walk up the escalator or take the stairs.

THIGHS

SMOOTH, firm thighs are not solely the preserve of models and exercise fanatics. Nor, are they likely to be the boast of a couch potato. You want them to look good. What is more, hormonal programming and the musculature of the thighs predispose them to gather fat. And fat, unfortunately, encourages wastes and fluid to accumulate, often resulting in cellulite, which is both unhealthy and unsightly.

COMMON PROBLEMS

- Loose and solid cellulite – sluggish circulation and hormonal imbalances cause fat and toxins to collect and become trapped in waterlogged tissue on our thighs. A sedentary lifestyle, poor muscle tone and a diet high in processed and refined foods are all significant contributing factors.

- Dry skin – due to poor circulation and a build-up of dead cells. Although thighs are subject to friction, dead cells are not evenly shed. This can make the skin texture and pigmentation appear uneven.

- Flabby thighs – lack of exercise, or failure to maintain exercise after upper leg muscles have been worked, causes thighs to become heavy and shapeless. Our inner thighs are particularly vulnerable.

- Thread/spider veins – an inherited tendency which generally worsens with age. Superficial capillary walls remain dilated and therefore visible (especially under thin skin), due to hormonal changes or the topical application of steroid creams. Some may become damaged through injury.

What to Do

- Thread veins can be safely and painlessly eliminated using a mild electric current which cauterizes (that is – closes off) the damaged capillaries and stems the flow of blood. The alternative treatment is sclerotherapy, where a solution is injected to clear the blockage. Avoid very hot baths if you have thin, sensitive skin and a tendency to thread veins.

- For help with dry skin and flabby thighs, see relevant sections in help for cellulite.

Firm thighs require

energetic **maintenance**

CELLULITE: TREATMENTS THAT WORK

A multi-faceted regime including:

Daily Thigh-firming Exercises

■ Use the plié, a classic ballet posture, to work the muscles of the thighs. Place your hands on your hips and stand with your heels together and your toes pointing outwards. Breathe in and rise up onto your toes. Breathe out and lower yourself into a squatting position, making sure that your back is straight (*see* below). Do not go any lower

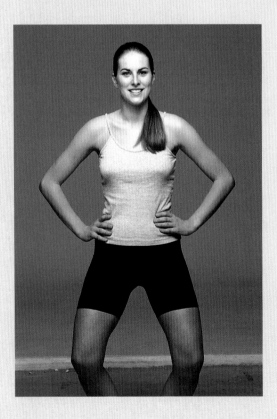

than is comfortable and stop if you feel any strain in your knees. Breathe in again and, pressing on the balls up your feet, raise yourself as slowly as you can to the standing position. Breathe out and rest. Repeat three times.

■ Sit with your back up against a firm surface, your knees bent and your fingertips resting on the floor beside you. Place a cushion between your knees, breathe in and, as you breathe out, squeeze the cushion between your inner thighs for a slow count of eight. Repeat five times. Make sure your inner thighs are doing the work while the other parts of your legs are relaxed.

■ Sit with your back up against a firm surface, the soles of your feet together and your hands lightly grasping your ankles. Breathe in and, as you breathe out, release your knees towards the floor. It sometimes helps to tuck a couple of plump cushions under-neath your knees so that there is something for them to relax into.

■ Brisk walking, rebounding (bouncing on a mini-trampoline), swimming and cycling are highly recommended for toning the big leg muscles. Rebounding is a great weapon in the battle against cellulite and one of the easiest forms of exercise to squeeze into a busy life.

Nourishment without Overload

- Eat plenty of fresh fruit and vegetables (organic when possible), wholegrains, pulses, fish and chicken.

- Kick-start the internal cleansing process with a raw fruit, vegetable or juice fast (*see* page 158).

- Eliminate wheat and dairy products for a three-month period to clear internal congestion (*see* page 158).

- Drink eight to ten glasses of water daily.

- Cut right back on your consumption of coffee, tea, fat, sugar, salt and alcohol, as they can disturb the body's internal balance.

- Avoid processed and refined foods – they contain very little nourishment and are usually loaded with additional salt, sugar and fat.

Massage

The objective is to pep up the circulation, disperse fatty deposits and encourage the drainage of excess fluid and waste via the lymph. Be patient – it has taken time for the excess baggage to accumulate and it will take time to eliminate.

- In a standing position, grasp handfuls of flesh between your thumb and all four fingers. Now 'pinch' all over your thighs, starting just above your knees and moving in the direction of your groin. Repeat the action on the backs of your thighs by resting your foot on a chair or the edge of the bath. Go easy if your skin has a tendency to bruise easily. Now massage the front of each thigh with the balls of your fingers, using small circular movements.

Dry Skin Brushing

Dry skin brushing with a natural bristle brush before your bath or shower boosts peripheral circulation and aids the flow of lymph while exfoliating the skin, which provides trapped toxins with another easy exit. Always brush in the direction of the heart and avoid broken or sore areas of skin. Alternatively, exfoliate your thighs energetically using the All-purpose Oatmeal Scrub (see page 36), on alternate days at first, then decreasing with improvement.

Mechanical Lymphatic Drainage Boots

These surgical thigh boots allow you to lie back while intermittent waves of pressure massage the lymphatic vessels in your legs, speeding up the removal of fluid wastes from the overloaded thighs. This treatment is only available in clinics.

Regular Salt Baths

Sea salt baths detoxify the system and regulate the fluid balance – essential steps towards reconditioning your thighs (*see* page 36).

Bikini Line

We all have a covering of fine hair on our thighs which does not usually bother us until the summer months. The problem can be made much worse by the friction caused by clothes and tampering – shaving and self-waxing – which often results in distortion of the hair follicles and problems such as spots and ingrown hairs. What to do:

■ Leave the area well alone or seek the help of a reputable therapist, if you think you need it.

■ If you decide to have electrolysis, opt for the non-invasive method such as scanning or the TE system (*see* page 70) in preference to needle methods, which carry a risk of scarring.

■ Exfoliate the area regularly to encourage healthy skin function.

CALVES AND SHINS

The blood vessels in our lower legs are engaged in a constant struggle to return used blood to the heart against gravity and deliver a regular supply of fresh blood to these outposts of the body. While this is happening, the lower leg muscles, which also play a part in this, are constantly in action, whether we are sitting, standing or walking, for example. Blood vessels and muscles are thus put under a great deal of strain.

COMMON PROBLEMS

■ Dry skin – due to reduced output of sebaceous glands, poor circulation, sun damage, ill health or as a side effect of medication.

■ Poor muscle tone – gradual loss of tone is usually caused by disuse, but well-developed calf muscles can also drop if they are not worked regularly.

■ Varicose veins – circulatory problem involving the failure of the valves in the deep veins of the lower legs. May arise from hormonal changes during pregnancy and the menopause, which cause the blood vessels to dilate and relax. Exacerbated by constipation, inactivity, excess weight, standing too long and hot weather. This condition is often hereditary.

■ Cellulite around the large calf muscle – caused by sluggish circulation which allows fluid and toxins to accumulate. Quite common during the menopause.

WHAT TO DO

■ Activate the acupressure points Spleen 6 and Stomach 36 to soothe pain, improve circulation and increase mobility in the lower legs.

■ To combat dry skin, grease yourself with almond oil before a bath and apply body lotion afterwards.

Exercise

The following massage will improve circulation in the lower legs and help to condition the muscles. It also provides welcome relief for tight, overworked calf muscles:

■ Place your feet flat on the floor and, using all four fingers, stimulate the back of the lower legs with a light 'pinching' action. Rest one ankle on the other leg and use your thumb to press and glide up the inside of the shin bone.

■ Apply the same technique with the index finger on the outside of the bone. Repeat the sequence on dry skin once a day if possible, reducing to once a week with improvement.

If you suffer from varicose veins, ignore the above routine and try stroking the lower leg from ankle to knee using the palms of your hands, lightly skimming over the affected area.

To Prevent or Relieve Varicose Veins:

■ Put your feet up at the end of the day (and any other moment you get the chance), to assist the return of blood to the heart. The feet need to be raised above the level of the head for at least 15–20 minutes to be really effective. Brisk walking to contract the leg muscles will also help to push the blood in the right direction.

■ It is a good idea to wear support tights when you are going to be standing for long periods. Also, train yourself out of crossing your legs, as this further impedes the circulation.

■ Controlling your weight and avoiding constipation are important safeguards.

■ Take a daily supplement of vitamin E.

■ Reduce your consumption of refined, sugary foods and step up your intake of whole-grains and fresh fruit and vegetables. Citrus fruits (skins and pulp), apricots, grapes, blackberries, cherries, broccoli, avocados, nuts, seed oils and buckwheat all help to strengthen and improve the elasticity of blood vessels.

FEET

'Out of sight is out of mind' seems to best describe our relationship with our feet. Our feet are designed for the unglamorous task of bearing our load which seems to give them a status inferior even to our hands. Given their long years of hard service, they ought instead to be pampered at every available opportunity.

The muscles of the feet also need to be worked or exercised regularly, otherwise they can no longer provide the necessary underpinning for the bone structure of the feet – or, for that matter, for the rest of the body – and problems start to occur.

> Our feet are furnished with a multitude of nerve endings and house a network of reflexology zones. These correspond to the different organs, glands and structures of the body (*see* right). The **reflexology zones** are stimulated as we apply pressure to different parts of our feet when we walk, unless the reflexes are blocked by hard skin or congestion. A systematic foot massage therefore has benefits which extend well beyond the immediate area.

The skin on the soles of our feet is thicker than anywhere else on our body and often becomes dry and hard. This is a natural consequence of the reduction in moisture levels which accompanies the ageing process, but mostly it's the skin's response to uneven pressure inflicted by ill-fitting shoes, worn-down soles and heels. It can also result from continually wearing high heels, which throw the weight forwards onto the balls of the feet. Try to vary the heel height of your shoes so that different muscles are pressed into action. It is also worth having your feet re-measured periodically as feet spread (and therefore increase in size) with age.

These are some of the problems I see:

COMMON PROBLEMS

- Hard skin and calluses – inappropriate footwear, the effect of poor posture and general wear and tear on the feet cause protective layers of skin to form. These become very thick and leathery if the underlying cause is not addressed and the feet not properly cared for. Excess weight adds to the problem by preventing the dead cells on the soles from being shed in the normal way.

- Dehydration – this is generally caused by the natural fall in the skin's moisture levels or by a dry skin condition. When feet are encased in a thick layer of dead skin which then becomes dehydrated, it can result in cracking and bleeding.

- Smelly feet – when the pH balance of the skin is disturbed, due to internal causes, which creates ideal conditions for bacteria to breed on the feet.

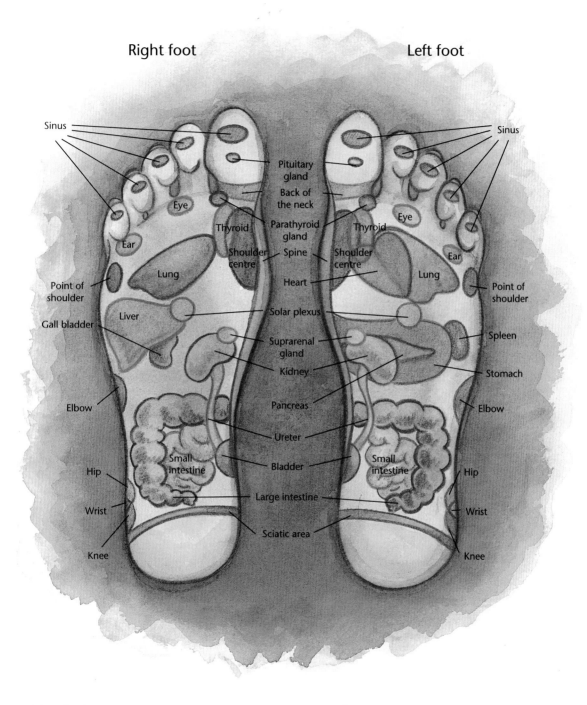

Right foot

Left foot

Sinus

Sinus

Pituitary
gland

Eye

Back of
the neck

Thyroid

Parathyroid
gland

Eye

Thyroid

Shoulder
centre

Spine

Shoulder
centre

Ear

Ear

Heart

Point of
shoulder

Lung

Lung

Point of
shoulder

Gall bladder

Liver

Solar plexus

Spleen

Suprarenal
gland

Stomach

Kidney

Elbow

Pancreas

Elbow

Ureter

Hip

Small
intestine

Bladder

Small
intestine

Hip

Wrist

Wrist

Large intestine

Knee

Sciatic area

Knee

The reflexology zones.

129

What to Do

You may never have beautiful feet – very few people do – but you will certainly have healthy, respectable feet if you follow this general advice:

> Soak your feet regularly in a **salt bath** (*see* page 22) to improve circulation in the feet, reduce the build-up of dead cells and control bacteria. The salts will also help to disperse any waste build-up in the delicate joints, thus protecting the stability of your feet.

■ Exfoliate your feet as often as you need to using an abrasive scrub. This will refine the skin and disperse any stagnated pigmentation around joints and other pressure points. Really leathery patches of hard skin may also need to be tackled with a pumice stone after soaking.

■ Follow up with a good foot cream (ideally with anti-bacterial or anti-fungal properties) or almond oil, massaged into the soles of the feet.

■ Give your feet a weekly massage treatment following the guidelines in Home Therapy (*see* page 15). This is a very effective way of reviving weary feet

which also guarantees a good flow of blood to nourish the skin and nails.

■ If your feet are suffering from long-term neglect, the above routines may be carried out daily.

■ Stick to natural fibres on your feet and expose feet to the air for a short period each day. Go barefoot whenever you can.

TOES

We ask very little of our toes and do virtually nothing in return. We overlook their basic need for air and space and quite forget that each of our toes has the potential for independent movement. Small wonder that they throw up more than the odd complaint.

COMMON PROBLEMS

■ Cuticle problems – an accumulation of dead cells causes the cuticle to become stuck to the nail at the base, so preventing the live part of the nail from 'breathing'.

■ Thickening of the nail – this occurs naturally as we advance in years. Other possible causes are psoriasis or fungal infection.

■ Ingrown toenails – a result of ill-fitting shoes and incorrect cutting and filing.

■ Corns and calluses – the appearance of hard skin due to friction is the body's way of protecting itself. These are more common in old age, when the fatty padding on our feet decreases.

■ Hairy toes – darker hairs do sometimes appear on the toes and can be very conspicuous. Generally more common in darker skin types. Friction created by footwear or hormonal imbalance may cause an increase in the diameter of normally fine hairs on toes.

■ Chilblains – a result of poor circulation, the skin on the tips of the toes becomes itchy and inflamed in cold weather. Aggravated by smoking.

■ Athlete's foot – a fungal infection caused by an imbalance in the pH of the skin and poor foot hygiene. Thrives on warm, damp skin. Most likely to occur when we are run down or after a course of antibiotics.

What to Do

■ Stimulate the circulation to the small joints in the toes by massaging each of your toes between your index finger and thumb. Continue for one or two minutes per toe.

■ Remove hard skin on top of bony areas with a pumice stone or an abrasive scrub after soaking.

■ Clip and file the nails squarely, in line with the end of the toes, so that the growth does not head into the surrounding soft tissue. File them regularly to avoid jagged edges. If you catch your nail, it can lift the nail, doing permanent damage to the nail bed and causing the nail to become deformed. Take care to keep the surrounding skin supple.

■ Remove hairs from toes by waxing, as this can help to weaken growth.

■ Spread and wiggle toes in the bath to liven up inert feet (your toes may not obey your commands to begin with). While soaking your feet, gently push back cuticles with a flannel, using small circular movements. Rubbing the toes with a flannel will also help to inhibit hair growth. Make sure you always dry toes thoroughly to avoid infection. Encourage children to do all these things as part of their bathtime routine.

Nourish the skin after a bath using a good anti-bacterial and anti-fungal foot cream (particularly if you suffer from athlete's foot) or almond oil. This will help corns and calluses and also improve your foot hygiene.

■ Massage the following acupressure points twice daily, Liver 3 and Urinary Bladder 60 (*see* pages 30 and 34).

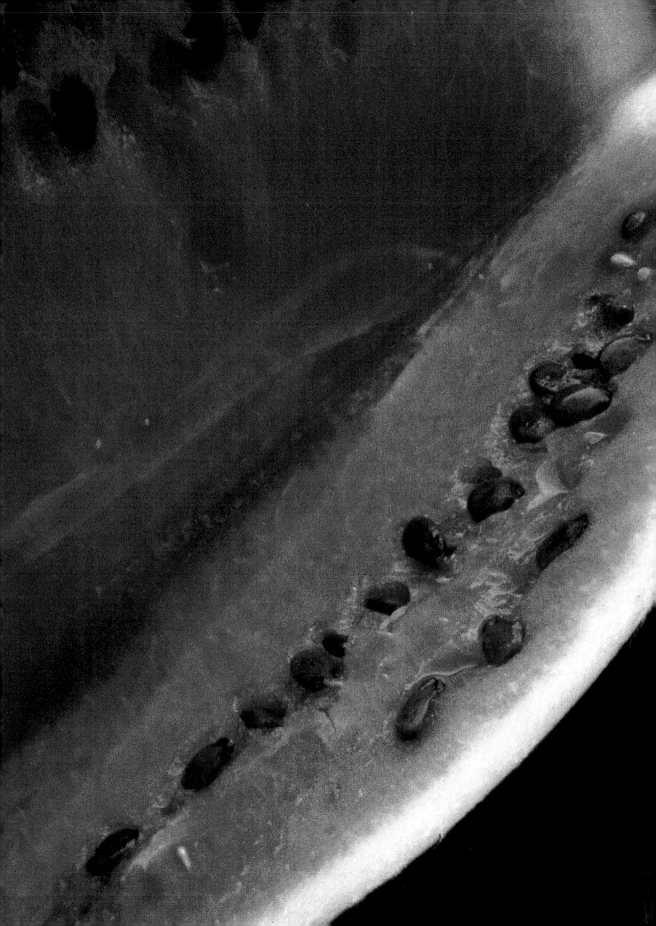

INNER HEALTH

BEAUTIFUL SKIN

WHAT IS SKIN?

PRACTICALLY speaking, our skin provides a protective waterproof covering for the contents of our body. It insulates us from the cold and lets off steam when we become overheated. It acts as a barrier against sunlight, potentially damaging germs and all manner of external pollutants, while excreting a proportion of our internal waste through its pores. In fact, the skin is the body's largest excretory organ, which steadily and continuously offloads waste as well as moisturizing the skin naturally – from the inside.

The skin is a living organ that breathes in oxygen and gives off carbon dioxide, as well as reproducing, nourishing and repairing itself using the raw materials made available by the body. Clearly, in order to understand and care for our skin properly, we need to have a basic grasp of what it does and how it is put together.

THE SKIN WE SEE

The skin that we can see is the upper surface of the epidermis, sometimes referred to as the stratum corneum. This consists of between 25 and 30 compressed layers of hardened skin cells, covered by a slightly acid and salty film. Composed of oily sebum (*see* below), sweat and a waxy substance called keratin, it is what is known as the 'acid mantle', which guards against invasion by bacteria and water loss via evaporation. This top layer of dry, dead cells is naturally worn away at the rate of 10 billion cells every 24 hours, to be replaced by a never-ending succession of new cells pushing up from the basal layer of the epidermis.

THE SKIN WE DON'T

Scattered liberally about the lower region of the epidermis are the pigment cells responsible for our skin colour and the tanning process, one of the body's natural defence mechanisms. Sunlight triggers the production of the brown melanin pigments and these spread through the epidermis, shielding the basal layer and underlying dermis from the harmful effects of the sun's rays. Pigment cells are also found in the deepest part of the hair follicle.

Skin is the *protective*

cover for our bodies

NUTS AND BOLTS

Beneath the epidermis lies the dermis, which provides the invisible but indispensable underpinnings for the visible top layer of skin. It acts as the skin's mattress, in the sense that its close weave of fibrous collagen and stretchy elastin fibres provide structure, support and resilience for the epidermis, as long as they remain in good condition. However, if these components are allowed to deteriorate, the skin is liable to sag and wrinkle. The proliferation of blood and lymphatic vessels – which supply the necessary nourishment and oxygen for collagen and cell production, and dispose of cellular waste – also play a vital role (*see* page 166).

The dermis is richly supplied with nerve endings which act as sensors for temperature, touch and pain. Also encompassed within the dermis are our sweat glands which, like the sebaceous glands (*see* below), adjoin our hair follicles. Virtually our entire body is covered with hair of varying thickness.

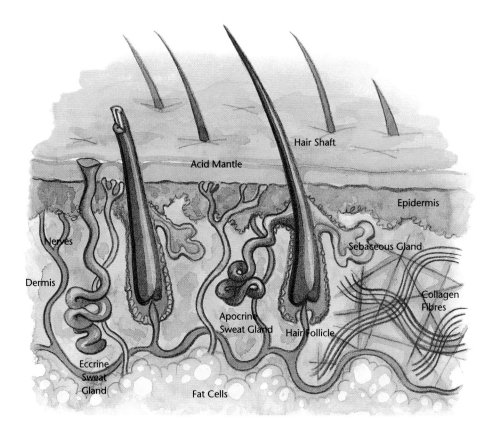

Cross section of the skin.

NATURAL OILS

The sebaceous glands are sac-like structures which open into the hair follicles and, via our pores, onto the surface of the skin. They secrete an oily substance called sebum, which helps to lubricate the skin and hair shafts. They are most numerous on our scalp, face, chest and upper back. Sebum offers protection against external drying elements such as the sun and central heating, for example, which is vital for the wellbeing of the skin and its appearance.

These glands remain quiet and unobtrusive throughout our childhood but suddenly spring into action at puberty. They continue to be pretty active throughout adolescence, giving rise to blackheads and acne, for example. Although over-production can be a problem, sebum is a valuable skin conditioner, and the oily skins of youth often turn out to have a head-start in the suppleness stakes later in life. An under-supply of sebum causes the skin to become dry and flaky.

MUSCULAR MAINSTAY

Lying independently beneath the skin or, in the case of our face, attached to the underside of the skin, are our muscles. The condition of our muscles has a huge part to play in the condition of our skin. Healthy muscles are relaxed enough to allow blood and waste to flow freely through them and firm enough to give shape to the flesh and hold the skin taut.

The Value of Fat. Fatty padding contained in the subcutaneous tissue, situated between our skin and our muscles, provides us with an insulating layer and a ready store of energy, as well as giving our bodies their womanly contours. Slightly overweight, mature women retain a fuller figure to their advantage. Stringent diets, prompted by excessive concern about weight gain in later years, may conversely lead us to diminish this cushion of fatty tissue, so valuable in plumping up the skin against progressive crumpling and creasing and boosting oestrogen levels after the menopause.

PROBLEM SKINS

SPOTS OR MILD ACNE

These problems develop when the sebum 'plug' which blocks the hair follicle becomes infected by bacteria that usually live harmlessly on the skin – itself an indication that the skin's acid mantle is out of balance – causing the sebaceous glands to become inflamed. Attempts to de-grease the skin with harsh cleansers and toners often aggravate the problem by stimulating sebaceous activity and so further disturbing the skin's protective covering.

If you suffer from recurrent acne, you will probably have been told by your doctor whether it is caused by a hormonal imbalance and may have been prescribed medication. While it is essential to work with your doctor to control any infection, you should be aware that any medication you do take will have some side-effect within the body, such as the disturbance of the friendly bacteria in the intestines by antibiotics, for example. There is also a danger that the body will become dependent if it is fed a synthetic version of the chemicals it should be producing itself, and further decrease its own output.

Your own habits can help to reduce the severity of attacks and the likelihood of cross-infection:

■ Affected areas need to be washed frequently with a pH-balanced soap and protected with a suitable moisturizer.

■ Apply the Healing Mask (*see* page 36).

■ Avoid handling, squeezing or picking spots at all costs.

■ Include plenty of fresh fruits, vegetables, wholegrains and live, natural yoghurt in your diet and try hard to maintain a regular intake of eight to ten glasses of water per day.

ECZEMA

An allergic condition caused by a deficiency in the immune system and characterized by dry skin and an

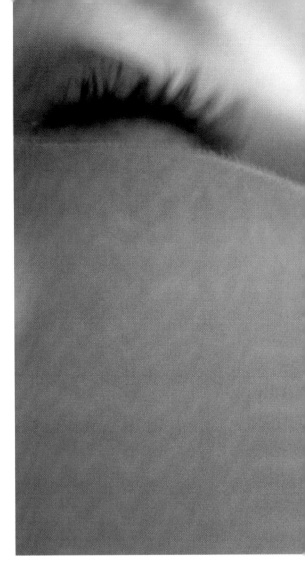

intensely itchy rash which is liable to blister and weep. Eczema is triggered by a baffling variety of sensitizers including foods, chemical substances, make-up, perfume, wool and stress. The pH balance is altered on eczema patches of skin, which means that they are easily infected and inclined to flare up.

■ Do some detective work to try to find the trigger for the outbreak. Watch your diet, being particularly aware of reactions to common food allergens

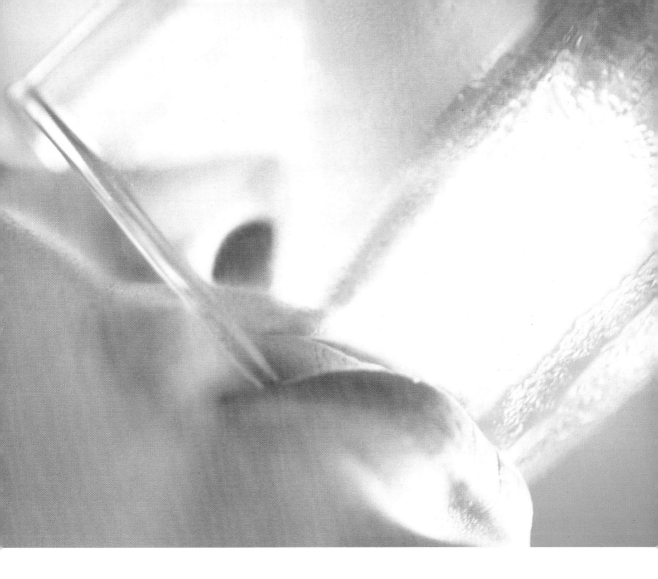

such as wheat and dairy products, citrus fruits, spices and alcohol.

■ Avoid all obvious sources of irritation.

■ Keeping the skin supple is a priority. Cleanse and moisturize regularly with liberal quantities of almond oil. Try an allergy-tested, tinted moisturizer or mousse foundation for camouflage purposes.

■ Soak affected areas regularly in Dead Sea salt baths (*see* page 22).

■ Use the Eczema Mask (*see* page 37), but do not rub or even use sponges to remove. Use once every week or fortnight on infected areas, depending on how irritated the skin is.

■ Beware of progressive skin-thinning caused by long-term use of steroid creams.

■ Drink plenty of water.

ACNE ROSACEA

A common condition, characterized by red, inflamed skin on the cheeks, nose and chin. Attacks are triggered in the highly sensitive mucous membranes of the nose, throat and sinuses in response to alcohol, spicy foods, extremes of temperature, hay fever or emotional stress, for example. If repeated or prolonged, they can result in the blood vessels becoming permanently enlarged. The condition often worsens around the time of the menopause.

- A corrective, green pre-foundation worn beneath your normal foundation will help to mask redness.

- Protect your face from the sun with a sun block or wear a hat with a wide brim.

- Drink eight to ten glasses of water religiously every day to dilute possible sensitizers in the bloodstream and flush out the facial tissues. If you do drink alcohol, make sure that it is with food and follow up with plenty of water.

- Gargle with warm salt water every morning to ensure that infection is not passed to your face via the throat.

- Do what you can to avoid unnecessary stress and anxiety. If you find yourself subject to unavoidable stress, a relaxing bath routine at least twice a week.

- Stimulate acupressure point Large Intestine 4 (*see* page 32) several times a day, to calm down the facial nerve.

- Cleanse and moisturize with almond oil or a little Vaseline, softened in the palm of your hand. Use the Stabilizing Face Mask (*see* page 36) once a week.

- Always handle your skin delicately. Massage your face and neck with a 'palming' action to calm irritated nerve endings.

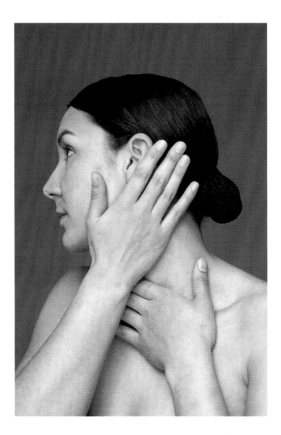

Skin Imperfections

- Liver spots – caused by cumulative ultraviolet radiation, these appear on the most exposed parts of the body in later years as a result of pigmentation changes beneath the skin. Refer to page 72 for help with this problem.

- Vitiligo – this absence of pigment in small, defined areas of skin can be caused by shock or stress, which produces a chemical that interferes with the function of melanin cells. It is also an occasional side effect of bleaching dark skins. Total sun block is essential to protect affected areas. Cosmetic camouflage can be very effective.

- Skin tags – small, greyish growths which usually appear on the neck and eyelids, but sometimes on the back and midriff. These often accompany the hormonal change in middle age and can be treated painlessly and successfully with high current electrolysis.

- Moles – these small, raised clusters of pigmented cells beneath the skin develop during adolescence and are mostly inconspicuous and trouble-free, although facial moles with protruding hairs can cause problems if the follicle becomes irritated and inflamed. Laser treatment is an effective method of removing moles which does not leave a scar. Consult your doctor, however, before having moles removed or if unusual-looking moles appear or a long-standing mole starts to change its shape or increase in size.

- Warts – caused by an infectious virus which invades the skin via tiny cracks and fissures resulting in abnormal growth of skin cells. They occur on the hands, knees, feet (the inward-growing verrucas) and on the face. Wait for warts to disappear of their own accord, treat homoeopathically or buy a suitable preparation at a chemist.

OUR CHANGING SKIN

From our mid-twenties onwards, changes start to take place in our skin which eventually cause it to lose its smooth texture, firm tone and uniform colour. This is what is referred to as the ageing process. The most significant changes, with far-reaching implications, are to the collagen and elastin fibres in the dermis. Due to a natural phenomenon called 'cross-linking', the normally pliable and well-ordered collagen fibres become rigid and disordered and lose their ability to stretch.

Falling moisture levels and dwindling supplies of elastin compound the problem as the collagen hardens still further and the skin's support structure collapses, causing wrinkles to appear where the skin would once have been held taut. In addition, reduced blood-flow deprives the cells of vital nutrients and encourages waste build-up at a stage of life when cell reproduction and turnover is already on the wane.

This speeded-up picture of skin deterioration and degeneration sounds rather alarming. In fact, the process occurs gradually over the space of several decades, at a pace broadly determined by your genes. However, it can be hastened or arrested by a number of factors, including sun damage, smoking, poor diet, stress, lifestyle abuse and misguided skincare or skin neglect, which *are* in your power to influence.

An additional and inescapable part of the ageing equation – and a law unto themselves – are **free radicals**, natural by-products of metabolism, but also released as a result of exposure to ultraviolet radiation, atmospheric pollution and smoking. These destructive 'loose cannons' hurtle about the body, destroying cell structures, sabotaging cell mechanisms and triggering chain reactions that undermine the fundamental ability of cells to reproduce healthy replicas of themselves. They also accelerate the degeneration of the tissues and are prime suspects in cases of premature ageing. But don't panic – you *can* arm yourself against them (*see* Amazing Almond Oil, page 150 and Suncare, page 152).

SAVE YOUR SKIN

So much is now known about how the skin works and there are many ways of helping to redress the effects of the ageing process. No one can delay this process indefinitely, but your skin does not have to show your age if you adopt certain habits and put various routines into practice early enough. In my opinion, it is never too soon – or late – to start.

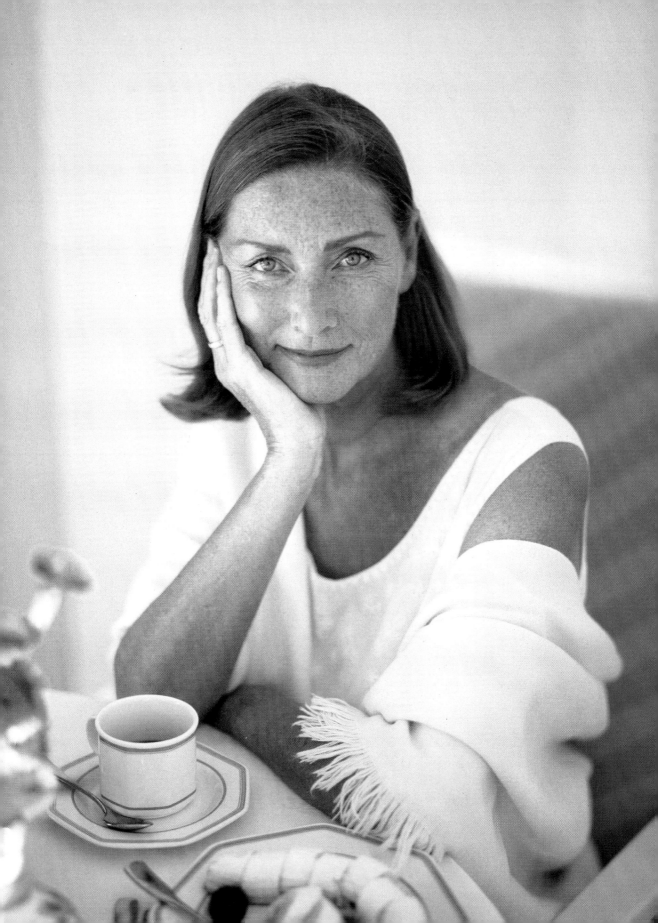

SKIN MAINTENANCE

The cornerstone of my healthy skin regime is regular massage following the face and body routines set out in Home Therapy (*see* pages 5–19). These movements are designed to condition the lower layers of the skin by improving the efficiency of the transport systems of the body – blood and lymphatic circulation – which carry nutrients and oxygen to the cells and waste material away from the tissues.

In order to be effective, these therapeutic routines need to be supported by sensible eating, drinking, sleeping, sunning and exercise habits. Thereafter, whatever you can do to boost the protective function of the skin and encourage the process of sloughing off and renewal, while minimizing moisture loss, will be to your advantage. This is where your skincare routine comes in.

The three pillars of skincare, whether you are dealing with your hands, feet, face or body are:

- Cleansing

- Moisturizing

- Exfoliation

CLEANSING

It may seem an obvious point, but keeping your skin clean is the number one skincare priority.

As the name suggests, **toners** have a mild (and short-lived) tightening effect on the skin. They are also great skin refreshers. Toners with a significant proportion of alcohol are described as astringents and should only be used on oily skins because of their drying action. They also have valuable antiseptic properties. Rosewater makes a freshening and fragrant tonic for dry and sensitive skin types. One of the best natural toners, however, is cold water. This can be splashed lightly onto your face – even your eyes – and directed at other parts of your body using a shower head, to bring fresh blood to the surface.

You need to cleanse your face both night and morning: in the morning to remove surface oil and dead skin cells after the night-time repair work to the skin has taken place, so that you begin the day with fresh skin; in the evening to remove the grime which has accumulated during the day and all traces of make-up. The morning routine need be no more than a swipe with a damp face cloth, but the evening cleanse should be extremely thorough. Any residue left on the skin slows down the repair process of the tissue and prevents the skin from 'breathing'. Remember: for cleansing purposes, your face starts at your collarbones and stops at your hairline.

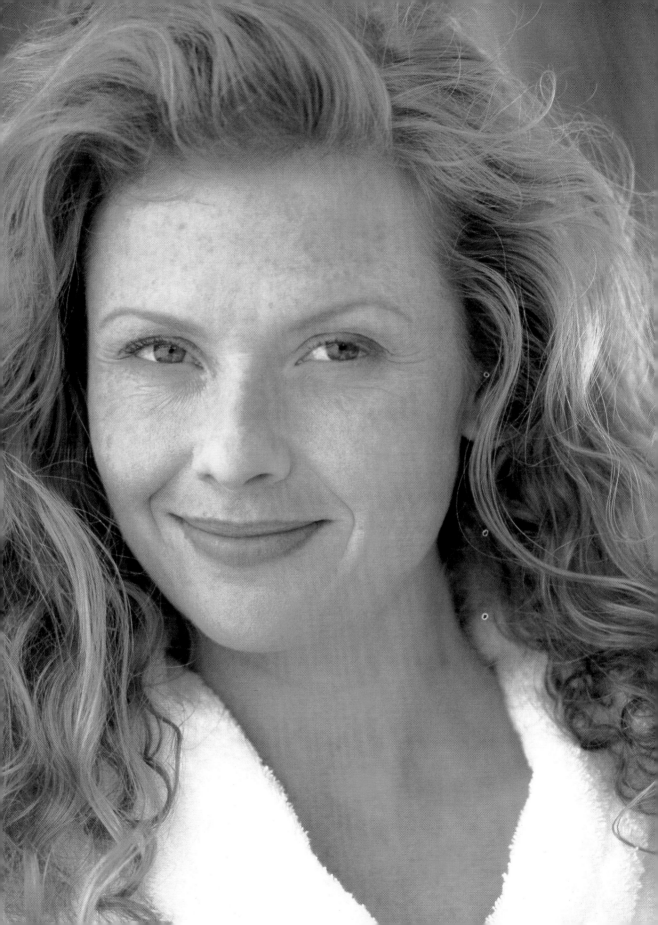

Sensible Soap

Washing with (the right) soap is one of the most effective ways of removing dirt and bacteria from your skin. Although most parts of your body do not require soap to get them clean, it is important to use soap in the areas of the body where sweat is prone to become trapped. People are frightened of using soap on their faces but, provided your skin is healthy and you moisturize properly afterwards, there is no reason to avoid it. The harm is done by harsh – that is, very alkaline – soaps, which disturb the skin's acid mantle, and the residue left as a result of insufficient rinsing.

- Stick to unadulterated soaps and those advertized as pH balanced.

- Only a smear is needed to do the job properly.

- Keep the washing process swift and efficient and rinse thoroughly afterwards.

- If your skin feels tight and uncomfortable after using soap, try one of the soap-free cleansing bars or foaming facial washes, or switch to a different type of cleanser altogether.

- Cleansing lotions, milks and creams are better suited to dry skins because they moisturize as they clean.

- To cleanse your nose properly, you need to cover the sides, stem, grooves and tip. If the skin on your nose is oily or congested, wrap a flannel around your index finger, lubricate it with a mild soap and, using small circular movements, go over the entire nose twice.

Traditional Tools. One of the oldest – and gentlest – methods of cleansing the skin, which cuts through surface grime and stale make-up without stripping the skin of its protective film, is oil. I am a particular fan of almond oil, but an unrefined vegetable oil, such as sunflower, is equally good. For sensitive and acne-prone skin, it is also a useful way to remove dead cells without irritation. I unreservedly recommend oil for mature skins.

Apply a light film of oil all over your neck and face, including your eyelids, and rub in gently using the balls of your fingers. Leave for up to a minute to allow it to work and remove with a dampened cotton wool or a facial sponge.

MOISTURIZING – A MUST

Our skin is equipped with its own natural moisturizer, a combination of sebum and sweat excreted all over the surface of our bodies via our follicles and pores. Moisturizing creams, which are basically oil and water emulsions, are based on the same ingredients, combined in varying proportions to create lighter/richer formulations. They should operate on the same principle, supporting this natural process and making up for any deficiencies. Some even incorporate constituents of sweat to increase their effectiveness.

The tendency to over-moisturize undermines the skin's capacity to keep itself taut. A simple analogy can be made with fabric conditioner applied to some washing: if you use the right amount, the clothes come out fluffy; too much makes them limp. You need to tap into your body's ability to work for itself. Allow yourself to be guided by the changing condition of your skin – and don't be frightened to leave it bare occasionally.

The basic function of a moisturizer is to maintain softness by keeping up the water level in the outermost layer of skin cells. It does this by creating a watertight seal which prevents what would otherwise be a continuous process of evaporation from the surface. At the same time, it provides a buffer to keep out potential 'invaders', thereby safeguarding the health of the lower regions of the skin, and ultimately the inner body.

- Get into the habit of applying oil or cream to slightly damp skin – night and morning – as this helps to 'lock in' valuable extra moisture.

- A layer of moisturizer creates a good base for and a barrier against make-up. Leave for 10 minutes and tissue off excess before applying foundation.

- If you are wearing a separate sunscreen, apply it *after* your moisturizer at least 15 minutes before going out into the sun.

Preventative Strike

As we get older, and the level of natural lubrication in our skin progressively diminishes, we compensate with creams, oils and moisturizing bath and shower preparations. It is not uncommon to experience a small crisis at this stage which leads us to step up the intensity of our skincare efforts instead of introducing the purest and simplest of measures, such as cleansing and moisturizing with almond oil, for example. This crisis – and the subsequent product overload – is less likely to occur if we take preventative steps and discourage dehydration by moisturizing our skin from an early age. Shielding the skin from sun damage from earliest infancy is also a vital part of this.

Never let your skin

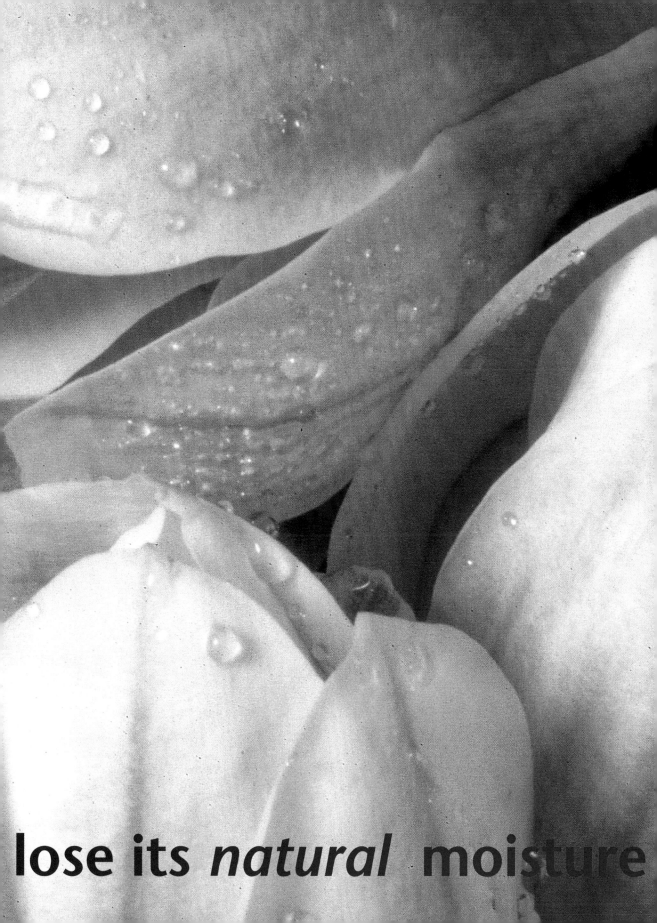

lose its *natural* moisture

Big Talk

Moisturizers are big business for the cosmetic companies, who are hard at work researching ingredients which might enable us to hang onto or recapture our youthful bloom. Today's products set out to achieve this by a variety of means: boosting surface protection with added ingredients such as antioxidant vitamins which control free-radical activity, sun protection factors, ceramides, phospholipids and collagen; delivering substances to the surface and the underlying layer to conserve and attract moisture and, in the case of the much-vaunted AHAs (or 'fruit acids'), having the capacity to stimulate the body's own moisturizing capabilities and collagen production.

In my view, the role of these products is limited and the claims made for them often exaggerated. What is more, the belief that one miracle ingredient can smooth out wrinkles or make good years of neglect leads people to go on trying one cream after another, with the result that their skin can become permanently irritated.

Amazing Almond Oil

Some of the mildest and most effective moisturizers are unrefined nut and seed oils, which gently soften and lubricate the skin and reinforce its protective film. The vitamin E and EFAs which they contain are invaluable for countering free-radical damage and strengthening cell walls. Almond (sometimes called 'sweet almond') oil is extremely well-suited to dry and sensitive skin. It can be used to moisturize every part of the face, including the eye area. Rub it into dehydrated skin before bathing or showering and pat yourself dry when you emerge – your skin will be left feeling supple without any superficial stickiness.

Aromatherapy-based preparations – plant essences in a base or 'carrier' oil – are some of the most deep-acting moisturizers, because of the capacity of essential oils to penetrate the skin and stimulate or regulate the activity in the tissues below. Make sure that the essential oils are pure and from a reputable source. The presence of free radicals in rancid oils will do your skin no good whatsoever, so buy in small quantities and keep bottles well-sealed and away from direct sunlight.

EXFOLIATE, EXFOLIATE

For our skin to remain clear, smooth and translucent, the surface layer needs to be kept free of any superfluous cells and its excretory activities able to continue unimpeded. That is why we exfoliate – to buff away the dead cells which otherwise might clog our pores and dull our complexion. There is an added incentive though.

The act of removing this redundant top layer appears to stimulate cell reproduction lower down in the epidermis – an increasing concern as our skin begins to age.

The danger, however, is that we do a lot more than is required to lift the unwanted dead cells, in the hope of bringing fresh cells to the surface faster. Instead, we undermine the barrier function of our skin and may even succeed in damaging the underlying tissue, with darker pigmentation marks and broken capillaries to show for it.

While it is important to curb any tendency towards heavy-handedness (think 'stroking' rather than 'scouring'), any skin will benefit from gentle exfoliation once a week to refine the texture and clear the pores. In addition, the massaging action flushes the skin with fresh blood and oxygen. Do not restrict your efforts to your face and neck. Callused feet, rough knees and parched elbows can be transformed by regular exfoliation, as can neglected hands and nails. Even areas of skin that appear to be smooth will attain a new height of silkiness once you have sloughed off the top layer of old skin.

- For a physical exfoliator or scrub, choose between a shop-bought product or a home-made preparation using a natural exfoliator such as oatmeal (*see* page 36).

- Apply the paste to damp skin and rub very lightly using circular movements.

- Moisturize your skin well afterwards.

- Newly exfoliated skin is more vulnerable to sun damage, so apply a sun block if you are going out in the sun.

- Dead skin cells which remain after bathing can be dislodged by rubbing your body lightly with a wet face cloth. You may prefer to use a mildly abrasive facial cleansing sponge or a soft muslin cloth to exfoliate your face.

- Moisturizing creams and toners (or clarifying lotions) containing AHAs exfoliate without extra effort by dissolving the glue which holds dead skin cells together. However, there is a risk of irritation with sensitive skins and multi-use of AHA products.

> **Facial masks** consist of a concentrated cocktail of active ingredients designed to deep-cleanse and revitalize the skin. The right mask can help rebalance problem skins, making them a very valuable addition to your skincare regime (*see* pages 36–37 for a list of recipes).

SUNCARE

Now that sunscreens are incorporated into moisturizing creams, foundations and powders, there is no excuse to lay yourself bare. For those serious about preserving the fragile skin on their face and neck, there is no better insurance policy than an application of SPF15 every day of the year. Antioxidant vitamins A, C and E – either in tablet form or applied to your face at night in an oil or cosmetic cream formulation – will further limit the free-radical damage.

- Choose a sunscreen that shields from UVA and UVB rays, and infrared if possible.

- Find yourself a wide-brimmed hat for alternative or additional protection.

- The latest physical (as opposed to chemical) sunblocks are unobtrusive enough to be used on your face and neck and are the sensible choice for sensitive skins.

- Apply your sunscreen half an hour before going out into the sun and top up regularly to maintain protection.

- Remember: hands and forearms are extremely vulnerable to sun damage, hence their tendency towards dehydration and liver spots. Apply sunscreen *as well as* hand cream during summer months.

- Areas of skin affected by an excess or loss of pigment need to be kept out of the sun or protected with a total sun block.

> **Wrinkle alert**. The toxins contained in cigarette smoke have a devastating effect on our respiratory system and skin. While our lungs silt up with tar, carbon monoxide monopolizes the oxygen-carrying capacity of our red-blood cells, which temporarily deprives our skin's cells of their vital supply. You can usually spot a smoker's skin: heavily (and prematurely) lined with a greyish, oxygen-starved complexion. If you are trying to give up, stimulate the acupressure points Heart 7 and Lung 9 whenever you feel the urge to light up (*see* pages 32–33). The general point, Lung 9, will restore the glow to smokers' cheeks and improve general vitality.

With every cosmetic house doing their best to persuade you to buy the latest 'miracle' products – creams and lotions for every part of the body promising to solve all your problems overnight – it is not hard to feel overwhelmed. And it can all get extremely expensive!

If you don't have the time to make your own kitchen cupboard treatments, it is important to know what to look for when you are buying skincare products. Here is a summary of recommended essentials:

- exfoliating cleanser to 'polish' the skin of your neck and face

- therapeutic oils to nourish the underlying tissues

- moisturizing cream with a high UV factor to protect your skin from sun damage

- rich moisturizer to bolster your skin in harsh winter weather

- moisturizing lotion for your body

- Dead sea salts for your bath

FEEDING YOUR BODY

THE food we eat provides us with the energy we need to live and the raw materials for the growth, maintenance and repair of our bodies. A regular intake of the essential vitamins, minerals, fibre, fats, carbohydrates and protein, together with water – in other words, a balanced diet – is all that it takes to keep the body's complex machinery ticking over. By supplying our bodies with these nutrients, we are also providing our skin, hair, nails, teeth, muscles and bones with the first-class nourishment that they require.

A healthy digestive system needs the support of efficient blood and lymphatic circulation to ensure that these life-sustaining raw materials are distributed throughout the body with sufficient regularity and also when they are at their freshest. Poor eating habits and digestive problems, however, undermine our general health and increase our susceptibility to illness. In a relatively short time, they can also have a visible impact on our appearance – most noticeably on the condition of our hair, nails and skin, for example.

BACK TO BASICS

WASTE DISPOSAL

Almost as important as the food we take in, is the swift and complete disposal of the waste products generated by our consumption. When these are retained as a result of constipation, the level of toxicity in our system increases. This is damaging to the body as a whole, but has particular repercussions for that often overlooked excretory organ, the skin. Poor elimination is a serious contributing factor in varicose veins, cellulite, premature lines and wrinkles and congested, spotty skin.

To combat or prevent constipation, step up your water consumption and intake of dietary fibre with plenty of fresh fruits and vegetables, wholegrains and pulses. This will assist the passage of undigested food through the gut. If you are unused to these foods, introduce them gradually. Other effective antidotes include regular exercise, avoiding refined, processed foods and building up your abdominal muscles (*see* page 115).

Valuable nutrients keep

skin and hair beautiful

WONDERFUL WATER

Nearly two-thirds of our body weight is made up of water. This is stored within the cells, outside the cells and in our body fluids. We *need* water to aid digestion and elimination. When we don't take in enough, toxins get trapped in our tissues, causing the complexion to deteriorate and laying the foundations for cellulite and the degeneration that heralds the start of the ageing process. So drink eight to ten glasses of water per day, ideally still-bottled or filtered.

Extract the juice from fruit and vegetables to enjoy their revitalizing and regenerating properties in a different form. The nutrients in freshly squeezed juice require very little digesting, so are absorbed more quickly by the body. For the best results, drink the juice immediately, sipping it slowly and holding it in your mouth for a few seconds before swallowing. A day or two on juice alone is a wonderful tonic to the system. Try your hand with oranges, grapes, papayas, mangoes and guavas (when in season), carrots, celery, grapes and ginger. Half a glass of freshly squeezed orange or carrot juice is an ideal way to start the day.

DEEP CLEANSE

Try not to allow wheat and dairy products to dominate your diet. Gluten, the gummy protein in wheat, and mucus-forming milk, cream, cheese and butter have a tendency to clog up the intestines and interfere with nutrient absorption. Tell-tale signs of congestion include a general feeling of sluggishness and an increase in the frequency of colds and other mucusy conditions. There is often expansion around the midriff too, not accompanied by weight gain elsewhere.

Excluding wheat and dairy products from your diet for three months will firm up and trim your figure, breathe new life into your skin and increase your general vitality, by improving your digestion and assimilation of food and keeping your respiratory system clear. It can take up to seven weeks to loosen the build-up in the intestines, which leaves five weeks or more for the therapeutic effects to be felt. In cases of very heavy congestion, a six-month period is recommended. Repeat every five years or so, as the need arises.

Wheat Products

Bread

Pasta

Most cakes and biscuits

Many breakfast cereals

Semolina, couscous

Bulgur (cracked wheat)

Wheatgerm and bran

Wheat Alternatives

100 per cent rye bread and crispbread

Rice (grains, cakes, noodles)

Potatoes

Oats (oatcakes, porridge, oatbran)

Corn (polenta, tortillas, cornflakes)

Buckwheat pasta and pancakes

Popcorn, pappadams, corn chips

Cornflour, potato flour, arrowroot
(thickeners)

Dairy Products

Milk

Butter

Some margarines

Cheese

Yoghurt

Dairy Alternatives

Goat's milk/cheese/yoghurt

Sheep's milk/cheese/yoghurt

Soya milk/yoghurt, tofu

Non-dairy margarine (*see* below)

Mayonnaise

Cold-pressed oils

Tahini

Hummus

THE BOTTOM LINE

The balance of your diet is clearly important. Although your appetite may tell you otherwise, your body needs a larger proportion of some types of food than others. There is also a great deal of evidence to suggest that a meat-free diet, or at least one that restricts our intake of meat, is an important step towards striking the right balance, by concentrating on foods that help the body to run more smoothly rather than adding to its burden. The following Daily Food Chart and Essential Nutrients section should point you in the right direction.

If you need to lose weight, a low-fat vegetarian diet is more likely to bring lasting results than a regime of deprivation, which ends up as a test of willpower that you are unlikely to win. Crash diets, although they might seem the answer to your prayers, can force your body to burn up precious muscle tissue which is later replaced with fat, as well as leaving a legacy of lines, wrinkles and loose skin unable to return to its former tautness.

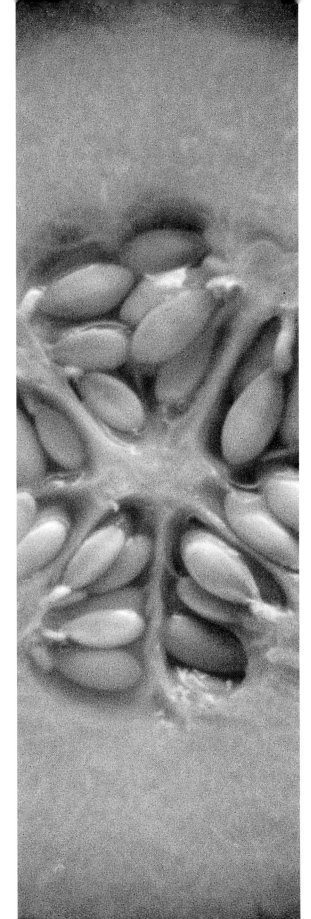

DAILY FOOD CHART

Here is a sample of a well-balanced eating plan to take you through the day, with recommended servings for each food type.

Bread/rice/pasta/cereal/potatoes

6 servings (e.g. 2 slices bread, 3 heaped tbs cooked rice or pasta, 90g cooked potato)

Fruit/vegetables

5 servings (e.g. small glass freshly squeezed fruit/veg juice, small mixed salad, 2 tbs steamed vegetables)

Fish/poultry/meat/eggs/nuts/seeds/pulses

2 servings (e.g. 75g oily fish, 300g cooked pulses)

Milk/cheese/yoghurt

2 servings (e.g. 200ml milk, small pot yoghurt)

Water

8–10 glasses

Fats

1 tbs 'good' fats and oils (*see* below)

THE ESSENTIAL NUTRIENTS

Carbohydrates

Supply energy needed for day-to-day running of body. Ideally, should make up half of your diet. Slow-burning, complex carbohydrates (fruit, vegetables and grains), eaten regularly, help to keep you on an even keel, both physically and emotionally. Choose wholegrains and unrefined cereals for maximum fibre and goodness, and try to eat a variety of cereals and grains.

Good sources

Breads, breakfast cereals, pasta, potatoes, rice, oats, rye, cracked wheat, buckwheat, millet, pulses, lentils, cornmeal, tortillas, corn on the cob, root vegetables, sweet potatoes.

- Choose oaty mueslis and cereals or porridge for a sustaining breakfast.

- Make salads using brown rice and cracked wheat as a base.

- Rye bread and loaves made of a mixture of grains make a change, as do soba noodles and buckwheat pasta.

- Incorporate rice cakes, oatcakes and rye crispbreads into snacks and light meals.

■ Use cornmeal for baking and to make polenta – a perfect accompaniment for grilled foods.

■ Cut down your intake of sugar as it is highly calorific, bad for your teeth and devoid of any nourishment.

Fruit and Vegetables

A vital source of vitamins, minerals, fibre and water. At least five portions a day recommended. These foods nourish and cleanse the body, but also protect it from disease. Vitamin C will strengthen collagen, capillaries and your immune system. Vitamin C, beta carotene (yellow-orange pigment found in carrots, apricots, mangoes, etc.) and vitamin E (in avocados and kiwifruit etc.) neutralize the effects of free radicals (see page 142). Potassium (contained in all fruits and vegetables) helps regulate fluid balance in cells and tissues and so combats fluid retention and bloating.

Good sources

Apples, apricots, artichokes, asparagus, aubergines, avocados, bananas, bean-sprouts, beetroot, broccoli, cabbage, carrots, celery, cherries, citrus fruits, cucumber, grapes, kiwifruit, leeks, lettuce, mango, melon, onions, parsnips, peaches, pears, peppers, pineapple, radishes, spinach, tomatoes, turnips, watercress.

■ Eat fruit and vegetables raw for their dynamic internal cleansing action and to maximize their food value.

■ Include a salad in most meals. Remember: *any* raw vegetables (or fruit) can be incorporated, there's no need to stick to tried-and-tested combinations.

■ Eat plenty of iron-rich spinach, watercress and parsley to keep up your haemoglobin level, particularly just before a period and during pregnancy.

■ Make fruit your staple snack food. Sweet fruits are a great source of instant energy – bananas are particularly sustaining.

■ Dark green vegetables are a good source of calcium for nails, teeth and bones.

Protein

Good sources

Lean cuts of meat, poultry, fish, milk, eggs, cheese, dried peas, beans, chick peas, lentils, nuts (unsalted), sesame/ sunflower/pumpkin seeds, cereals (especially wheatgerm), potatoes.

- Poultry and game contain less fat than other meats, plus the important B vitamins and iron. Avoid processed meats.

The body cannot carry out its vital functions without protein, but it only needs a modest amount to do so – around 55 grams per day. While hair, nail, teeth, collagen and muscle condition suffer when rations are short, they do not benefit from additional protein intake which, since it cannot be stored, is laid down as fat. Excessive consumption overloads the liver and kidneys – vital organs of detoxification – and can result in the loss of certain minerals, especially calcium, and an increased risk of osteoporosis.

- Fish is a great and healthy source of protein. Eat at least two portions a week. EFAs in oily fish and shellfish help to keep skin moist and strengthen hair and nails.

- Pumpkin, sesame and sunflower seeds are nutritional treasure troves packed with protein, fibre and many skin-saving and beautifying nutrients.

- Combine nuts and seeds, pulses and wholegrains for a highly nutritious cocktail of plant-based proteins, e.g. peanut butter/beans on toast, hummus and pittas. Pulses are an excellent low-fat, high-fibre source of protein.

Fats

- Use butter in moderation in favour of so-called 'healthy' margarines, loaded with additives, preservatives and poten- tially harmful trans fatty acids. With 'safe' margarines (labelled 'unhydrogenated') – the oils have not been subjected to the solidifying process that causes them to behave more like saturated fats.

- Buy soft cheeses and those made with sheep's and goat's milk. Substitute Quark for cream cheese.

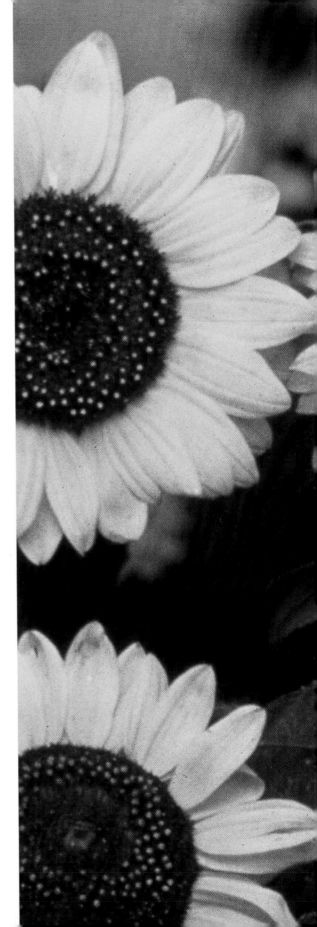

Fats are essential and should represent 30 per cent of food intake. A concentrated source of energy – and therefore calories – so choose carefully. Our bodies cannot work without fats which, amongst other things, are needed to absorb the fat-soluble vitamins A, D, E and K and provide protective padding for delicate organs and bony areas. Excluding fat, particularly the beneficial unsaturated variety, is bad news for your health and looks. Also, a clear link exists between heavy consumption of saturated fats (in butter, hard cheese and red meat) and heart disease. Strike the right balance by opting for reduced-fat dairy products and supplement with small quantities of health-enhancing monounsaturated and polyunsaturated fats (EFAs) found in avocados, olive oil, sunflower oil, nuts, seeds and oily fish.

■ Make sure that all the oils you buy are cold-pressed and unrefined – that is, nutritionally intact. Fry only with olive and sesame oil, as these remain 'stable' at high temperatures, but never heat to smoking point. Corn and sunflower oil can be used for gentle frying.

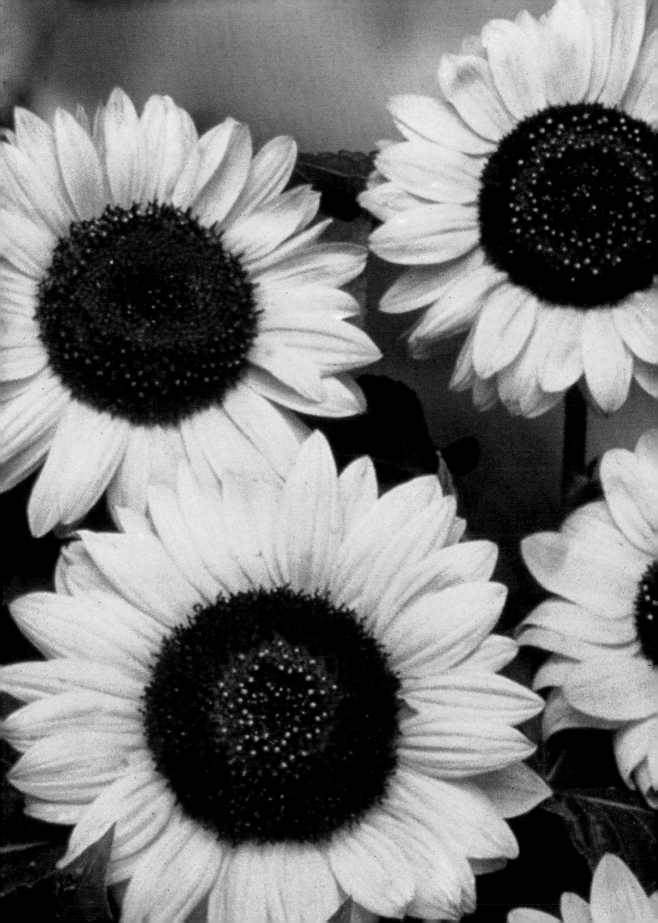

VITAL FLUIDS

Y OUR life depends on your body being able to deliver regular supplies of nourishment and oxygen to every tiny cell, and remove the rubbish which would otherwise pollute your tissues. We have in our heart and blood vessels both a powerful mechanism and an extensive circuit to achieve this, backed up by a network of neighbouring lymphatic vessels.

DRENCH AND DRAIN

The lymphatic system (which also maintains a fluctuating reserve of water in between the cells) acts as the skin's internal irrigation service, sluicing out potential pollutants and keeping the conditions in the tissues as salubrious as possible. The main drainage point for the lymphatic system is located in the groin, which is one of the reasons why we treat the face and body together: it helps to clear the system as a whole.

The lymphatic system works away in the shadow of the blood circulation, closer to the skin's surface. A network of tiny tubes hoovers up debris and leaked fluids from the spaces between the cells and conveys it to filtering stations, known as lymph nodes, which remove all the harmful wastes and bacteria. These eventually flow into the veins, enabling the missing fluids to be returned to the blood. In this way the lymphatic system plays a vital role in maintaining a healthy internal environment. However, since it relies on the massaging effect of the muscles and a good breathing action rather than a central pump to propel the fluid around the body, it is prone to become sluggish.

Fluid wastes are circulating around our systems all the time without necessarily doing any harm. It is only when they are allowed to settle in our tissues that they begin to wreak havoc. A state of affairs which is sometimes described as 'stagnation', when the resulting toxic sediment causes progressive deterioration of the tissue unless action is taken to disturb and dispose of it. Problems also arise if the amount of water required by the body for efficient circulation is drastically reduced, as it is by chronic constipation and crash dieting. Our face is particularly vulnerable to these problems due to the patchy coverage and precise configuration of blood vessels (*see* page 88).

The lymphatic system *rids*

MARVELLOUS MASSAGE

The good news is that we are able to boost our circulation and keep stagnation at bay on our face and our body with the help of gentle massage, which encourages lymphatic flow and drainage and so corrects any imbalances. Every little helps. Even the mild friction generated by the action of cleansing, moisturizing and exfoliating your skin spurs the circulation into activity. Repeating the Home Therapy routines on a weekly basis (*see* pages 5–19), will give your system a regular shot-in-the-arm. Remember, when your circulation is good, you flourish on the inside and glow on the outside. What is more, you can prevent many common problems occurring.

These are just some of the benefits of such massage:

- Transforms the condition of all skin types and increases the capacity of dry skin to absorb nourishment.

- Promotes firm, supple skin by providing regular nourishment for elastin and collagen fibres in the dermis. If these sensitive components are overloaded with toxins, they do not take what they require from the bloodstream.

- Limits the hormone-related damage caused by overactive sebaceous glands, by creating a clear channel for removal of excess sebum.

- Keeps the network of capillaries in good working order and helps curb tendencies such as broken capillaries or acne rosacea.

- Activates the cells which have become dormant to do their job properly – that is, encourages the skin's natural process of shedding and renewal.

- Improves lymphatic drainage around the eyes – the most common site of lymphatic blockage – and prevents the permanent discoloration sometimes caused by dark shadows.

- Maintains healthy joints by protecting the cartilage which surrounds them from damage caused by stagnation.

So start massaging. You will soon see the benefits.

So what bearing do these internal systems have on our external appearance? The answer is – considerable. It is impossible to radiate good health and good looks if our system is deprived of oxygen and nutrients or overloaded with toxins. Some of the beauty problems which arise from impaired or defective circulation of blood and/or lymph have been covered in Top to Toe, everything from poor skin, hair and nails to loss of muscle tone, cellulite, prematurely aged skin and varicose veins.

your body of toxins

Our hormones do an amazing job, fine-tuning the activities of our organs and life-support systems to maintain our internal equilibrium and health. Problems arise when the ebb and flow exceeds normal bounds or we introduce synthetic hormones into the body, creating hormonal imbalances which can disturb those internal mechanisms and affect the condition of our skin, our normal patterns of hair growth and pigmentation and the shape of our bodies, as well as inducing dramatic shifts and swings of mood.

The main triggers for hormonal imbalance are:

■ Puberty, pregnancy and the menopause

■ The fluctuations within the menstrual cycle itself

■ The contraceptive pill

■ HRT

■ Steroid-based medication

Hormones affect our appearance in the following ways:

■ An increased tendency to spots and acne caused by raised levels of androgens, which disturb the activities of our sebaceous glands.

■ The appearance of excess facial or bodily hair in women due to a surfeit or increased sensitivity to the androgens circulating in the blood.

■ Abdominal bloating, breast swelling and weight gain due to a high oestrogen /low progesterone balance; facial puffiness caused by long-term use of steroids.

■ Cellulite as a result of oestrogenic activity.

■ Darker patches of pigmentation caused by shifting oestrogen/progesterone levels during pregnancy, the menopause and as a result of taking the contraceptive pill.

■ Thinning hair and hair loss on our scalp reflect imbalances associated with menstrual irregularities, the pill, a fall in oestrogen and progesterone levels around the time of the menopause, HRT or thyroid problems.

Hormones affect our

THE EFFECTS OF STRESS

Stress which is not kept under control adds to the cocktail of circulating hormones and often intensifies their effects. It also interferes with the normal function of many of the body's vital processes, including our breathing, our digestion and our circulation.

Regular stimulation of 'sedative' and 'homoeostatic' acupressure points (*see* pages 28–35) and Dead Sea salt baths will prevent stress from getting the better of you.

Anxiety about spots in adolescence, accompanied by mental and emotional confusion as you experiment with different treatments, hoping to relieve the problem, but insufficiently informed to know how, is a classic example of stress turning a hormonal hiccough into hormonal chaos. In a situation like this, a practical skincare routine and proper relaxation is required to limit the damage. The hormonal impact of stress on your body can also make the difference between a smooth and a disturbed menopause.

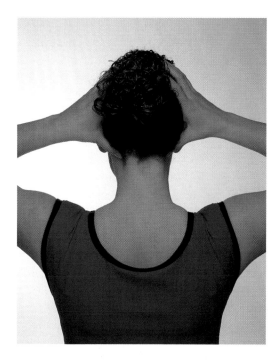

Embrace tears: they are a valuable safety valve and release mechanism which can help to diffuse an internal crisis without your hormones having to bail you out.

health and our mood

Our muscles are the flesh on our bones; they determine our strength and our silhouette. Beautiful muscles are healthy, firm and supple. Good muscle tone is important for our health and our looks, whether we are talking about the voluntary muscles that move our skeleton or the involuntary muscles that enable our internal organs to function. Muscle tone is what keeps the fleshy part of our muscles firm and effectual. When tone is lost, the muscle becomes less efficient and wastes accumulate (in much the same way that a pool of water collects beneath a tap which has not been tightened properly).

TAKING CONTROL

We need the control provided by well-toned, underlying muscles to keep our flesh taut. Whether you are super-lean or well-built, you will look and feel firmer and more compact if you maintain your muscle tone. There are other compelling reasons to prevent your muscle tissue from going to waste:

■ From middle age onwards, the body's balance of muscle to fat gradually tips in favour of the latter. This puts the onus on us to take preventative action sooner rather than later.

■ Since muscle tissue is metabolically active, the more muscle tissue you have, the greater your fat-burning potential.

■ The desire to redefine your contours, make your movements more graceful and economical, and add to your energy reserves.

Your face is swathed in muscles: long, straight ones covering your neck, cheeks and forehead; circular ones around your eyes and mouth; and a layer of deep muscles in your neck housing vitally important arteries, veins and nerves. Many of these delicate, interlinking muscles are attached to the skin (as opposed to being firmly tethered to bone as they are elsewhere in the body), which makes them vulnerable to damage from heavy-handed skincare routines and massage. So go gently.

Good muscle tone gives

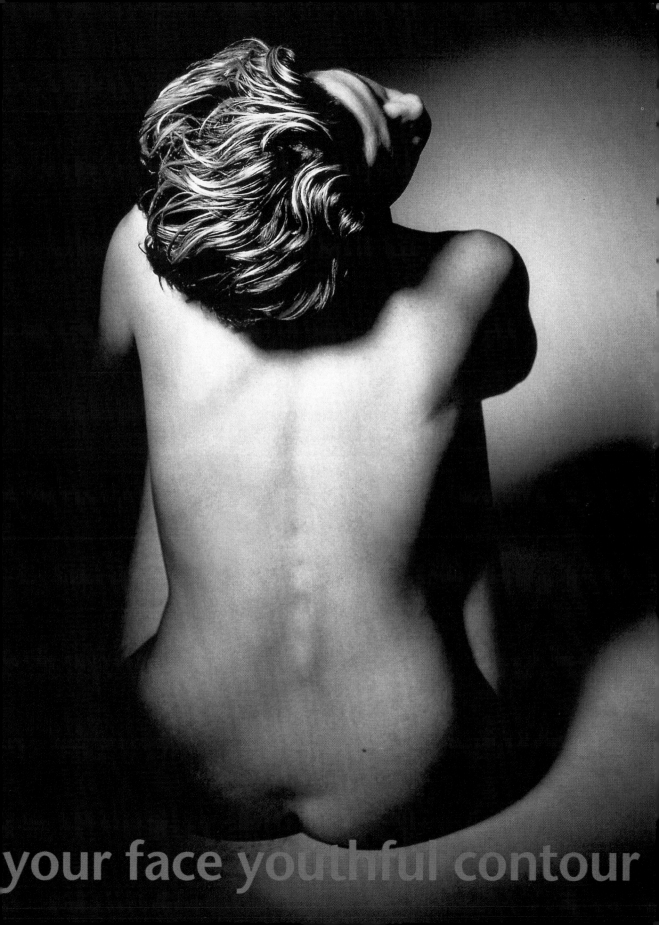

your face youthful contour

FACE FACTS

From our mid-twenties onwards, we experience a progressive and inevitable decline in the tone of our facial muscles, which can be softening on both the profile and the skin. If, however, these muscles become overburdened with waste or excess bulk, the deterioration can be swift and sudden, causing the flesh to droop and the skin to hang in folds. With the help of a targeted programme of exercise and massage (*see* pages 9–12, 60, 78 and 94), you can slow down the pace of deterioration and reclaim some degree of tone. The muscles around the mouth and eyes, in the cheek area and along the jawline are in greatest need of regular attention.

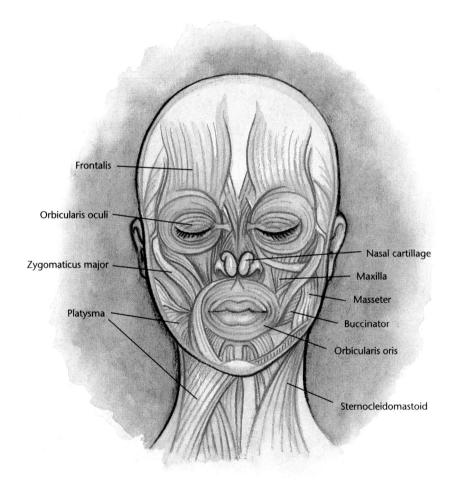

Frontalis

Orbicularis oculi

Zygomaticus major

Platysma

Nasal cartillage

Maxilla

Masseter

Buccinator

Orbicularis oris

Sternocleidomastoid

The Lion Pose

The following exercise performed once a day (in the privacy of your own home!) will stop your face and neck muscles from ever going into retirement.

■ Take a deep breath and, as you breathe out slowly, open your mouth as wide as possible and stick your tongue out as far as it will go. At the same time, look at the ceiling without raising your head or straining your eyes.

■ Maintain the position and count slowly up to 12. Aim for five repetitions.

BODY BEAUTIFUL

Elsewhere in the body it is generally the large muscles which give us trouble – the buttocks, fronts and backs of thighs, abdominal muscles, and, to a lesser extent, the upper arms – as when they are slack and out-of-condition, they have a powerful attraction for fat, fluid and toxins.

Effortless Exercise

Try to keep up regular aerobic exercise, but don't despair if you find this too difficult. You will be surprised by how much you can achieve with the simple routines outlined in Top to Toe. Many of the exercises can be done when you are on the move or going about your daily tasks. These exercises are intended to provide a basic framework so that you can create your own programme which addresses your particular needs. Add your own routines – any rhythmical movement that you enjoy will nourish and cleanse your muscles. If you like dancing, for example, do it whenever the mood grabs you.

Walk regularly. It keeps calf and thigh muscles active, and helps with the difficult task of pumping your blood and lymph back up the legs against gravity. This guarantees good lymphatic clearance and wards off varicose veins. Be aware of your upper and lower leg muscles working as you move along. Spring from one foot to the other and squeeze your buttock muscles to propel yourself forward.

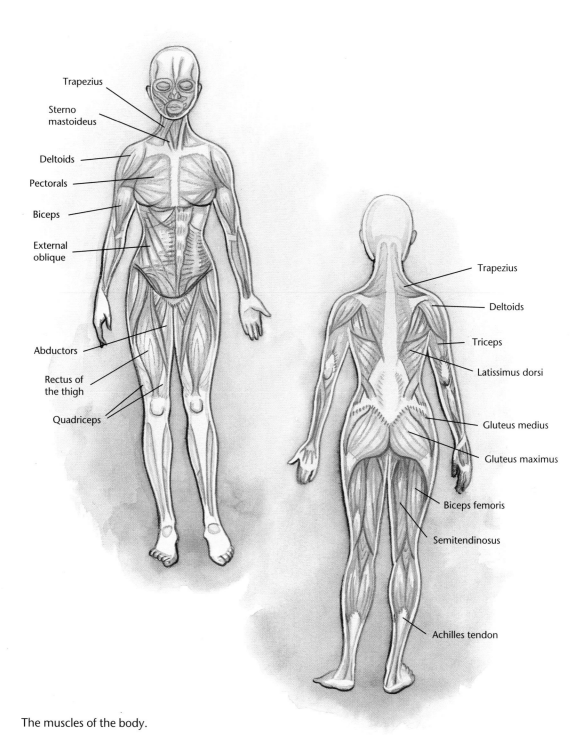

The muscles of the body.

HELPING HANDS

Massage is an easy way to promote muscle health. Using our hands, we can encourage the flow of nutritious, oxygen-rich blood into the muscles and stimulate the discharge of harmful wastes. By triggering a powerful activator present in every muscle, massage also has a remarkable ability to build up and restore muscle tone. Refer to Home Therapy (pages 5–19) for massage routines for the face and body.

BANISH TENSION

Tense muscles are a dead weight as far as the body is concerned and a drain on energy reserves. The discomfort we experience from chronically tense muscles is caused by the waste products which have become lodged within the muscles themselves. Over a period of time, such tension can result in raised blood pressure. Palming and pinching (*see* page 7) are both valuable massage techniques for unclenching contracted muscles and restoring them to full health. Pinching is also useful for shifting stubborn fatty deposits.

Facial tension is something which affects us all, even though we may not be aware of it. It can manifest itself as a tired, lifeless complexion or wooden, expressionless features, as though the muscles of your face had become frozen. Tapping with the balls of your fingers on your cheeks, across your forehead, around your mouth and even over your scalp is a gentle way of releasing locked muscles. The following acupressure points are also very effective in disolving facial tension: Large Intestine 4 and Taiyang (*see* pages 32 and 35).

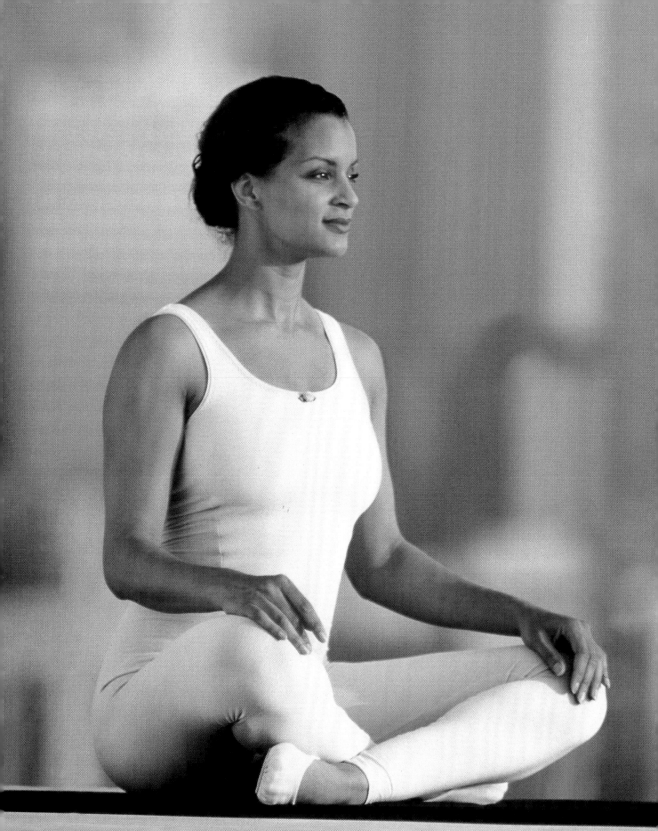

Deep *breathing* promotes

BREATHING FOR BEAUTY

Our need for oxygen is even greater than our need for water and food, as our cells cannot survive or function properly without it. Our respiratory system carries out the following vital functions:

- To draw the oxygen from the air into our lungs.

- To pass it on to the red blood cells, the 'couriers' that convey the oxygen to the cells.

- To eliminate carbon dioxide waste.

BREATHE DEEP

Good breathing uses the diaphragm – a sheet of muscle beneath the lungs and ribcage which flattens out to allow for a maximum intake of air. It is impossible to achieve if your posture is slumped or tensed. Try this experiment to see how you fare:

- Rest one hand on your tummy, around your navel, and place the other on your upper chest.

- Breathe slowly and deeply and watch where the movement is taking place.

When you are breathing well, most of the visible activity appears to be going on in your abdomen, which moves slowly in and out. Note how it feels and looks and contrast it with breathing (often triggered by anxiety) which involves rapid movements of the upper chest. Good breathing can calm and prevent anxious states.

THE BENEFITS

Good breathing, and for that matter good, clean air, floods our cells and tissues with dynamic oxygen which has the power to galvanize cell metabolism and boost cell turnover. The benefits are immediately noticeable in the freshness of our skin

Most of us take our breathing for granted. However, by focusing on our breathing, we can improve the flow of oxygen and prevent internal pollution, both of which have a dramatic impact on the way we look and feel.

fresh skin and bright eyes

tone and the brightness of our eyes. And, because everything is ticking over efficiently, we feel more alert and alive. Proper abdominal breathing helps to streamline the midriff and gives your frame underlying strength, discipline and poise. Steady, deep breathing also cleanses the system by increasing the output of potentially toxic, waste gas and providing some assistance to the lymphatic circulation.

> **Ginger** has a strong affinity with the mucous membranes that line the respiratory tract, and the ability to curb troublesome mucus production. The warming properties of ginger allow it to liquefy excess mucus, which keeps the passages of the nose and throat clear and helps indirectly conditions such as tinnitus. Ginger is also very effective in clearing the sinuses and even has the potential to reduce asthmatic tendencies.

OXYGEN FOR ENERGY

The body runs out of steam for many different reasons. Sometimes sleep is the only cure. More often, however, it is simply a question of the body's battery running low. One of the most effective ways to recharge your batteries is by concentrating on your breathing for five to ten minutes. This can be more refreshing than a nap and will not disturb your night-time sleep patterns or leave you feeling groggy. Do it either sitting or lying down:

- With eyes closed rest your hands on your abdomen and breathe in gently, pushing against your hands as you do so.

- Breathe out, lingering over the outbreath until the need for another inbreath naturally arises. Do not exaggerate the inhalation or the exhalation, in fact, the quieter the better.

- Continue to observe your breathing until this deeper, slower rhythm has become automatic. Stop when you feel your strength returning.

This is also a good technique for winding down and preparing to go to sleep at night.

YOGA

Exercise, in any form, intensifies all the benefits of good breathing. Yoga postures (*asanas*) are especially valuable because they teach you to become aware of your breathing and to use it as a means of relaxing, resculpting and revitalizing your body. When you are in a relaxed state, the oxygen level in your bloodstream is higher and your body is in balance. Proper relaxation also takes the pressure off all body systems and provides an opportunity for much-needed recuperation.

The breath control exercises (*pranayama*) that are part of yoga practice can be very invigorating. Wake up your system in the morning with these two routines and you will start the day with a radiant glow:

- Close your right nostril with your right thumb and inhale deeply through your left nostril. Close both nostrils and hold the air in your lungs for as long as is comfortable. Next, close your left nostril and exhale slowly through your right nostril. Keep your left nostril closed and inhale through your right nostril. Close both nostrils. Now slowly exhale through your left nostril. This is one cycle or round. Try to do three or four rounds each time.

- Now adopt a comfortable sitting position, placing your hands on your knees and lowering your eyes. Inhale and exhale quickly and forcefully, like a pair of bellows. Start with one exhalation per second and gradually increase speed. Aim to complete one cycle of ten exhalations initially and increase gradually.

The second exercise (*kapalabhati*) has many benefits. It clears the head, the nasal passages and the respiratory system. It brings huge supplies of oxygen into the lungs and draws out large quantities of carbon dioxide from the body, so purifying the blood. It also tones up your heart and activates the respiratory, circulatory and digestive systems.

Yawning is the body's clever way of delivering a huge blast of oxygen into the system. We yawn when we are tired or when our breathing becomes shallow due to stress or anxiety. Make sure you really luxuriate in the stretch – just follow the example of cats and dogs! You'll find that this also helps your muscles to relax.

Respiratory Tonic

Drink the following every morning on an empty stomach:

6–7 drops freshly squeezed ginger juice (peel a small ginger root, grate it and press it), $1/2$ tsp honey in half a glass of hot water.

FURTHER READING

Ball, J. *Understanding Disease* (C. W. Daniel, 1990)

Ballentine, R. *Diet and Nutrition: A Holistic Approach* (Himalayan Publishers)

Bennett, R. *The Science of Beauty Therapy* (Hodder and Stoughton, 1995)

Brostoff, Dr J. & Gamlin, L. *The Complete Guide to Food Allergy and Intolerance* (Bloomsbury, 1993)

Davis, A. *Let's Get Well* (Thorsons, 1992)

Earle, L. *Eat Yourself Beautiful* (BBC Publications, 1992)

Earle, L. *Vital Oils* (Ebury, 1991)

Gala. Dr D. R. & Gala Dr Dhiren *Care of the Eyes* (Gala Publishers)

Guyton, A. *Anita Guyton's Anti-Wrinkle Plan* (Thorsons, 1994)

Harrold, F. *The Massage Manual* (Headline)

Hutton, D. *Vogue Futures* (Ebury, 1996)

Imrie, Dr D. with Dimson, C. *Goodbye Backache* (Sheldon Press)

Kenton, L. *The Joy of Beauty* (Vermillion, 1995)

Kenton, L. *Passage to Power* (Vermillion, 1996)

Kingsley, P. *Hair: An Owner's Handbook* (Aurum Press, 1995)

Llewellyn-Jones, D. *Everywoman* (Penguin, 1993)

MacKie, R. M. *Healthy Skin: The Facts* (Oxford University Press, 1992)

Madders, J. *Stress and Relaxation* (Vermillion, 1997)

Meredith, S. *Eczema: A Comprehensive Guide to Gentle, Safe and Effective Treatment* (Element, 1994)

Nightingale, Dr M. *Holistic First Aid* (Vermillion)

Rama, S., Ballentine, R. & Hymes, A. *Science of Breath* (Himalayan Institute)

Reader's Digest *Foods That Harm, Foods That Heal* (Reader's Digest, 1996)

Sharma, Dr P. D. *Yogasana and Pranayama for Health* (Gala Publishers)

Smyth, A. *Thorsons Encyclopaedia of Natural Health* (Thorsons, 1997)

Young, J. *Acupressure for Health* (Thorsons, 1994)

PHOTOGRAPHIC ACKNOWLEDGEMENTS

THE publishers and authors thank the photographers and organizations for their kind permission to reproduce the following photographs in this book:

Page 2	TCL, by Kathy Collins
Page 20	courtesy of Finders
Page 22	courtesy of Finders
Page 24/5	TS, by Chris Craymer
Page 40	TCL, by Daniel Kron
Page 43	TS, by Andre Perlstein
Page 51	TCL
Page 67	TCL
Page 76	TCL
Page 93	TCL
Page 98	ICL, by P. Sancho
Page 103	TS, by Nick Dolding
Page 105	TCL, by Sarah Hutchings
Page 107	TS, by Bernard Pesce
Page 117	TS, by Nick Dolding
Page 123	TCL, by Paul Viant
Page 135	TS, by Claude Guillaumin
Page 138/9	TCL, by JP Fruchet
Page 143	TCL, by Nick Clements
Page 145	TS, by Daniel Bosler
Page 156	courtesy of Finders
Page 162/3	courtesy of Thompson and Morgan
Page 167	Oliver Hunter
Page 169	TS, by Stephanie Rushton
Page 174	TS, by Lori Adamski Peek

Key
TCL: Telegraph Colour Library/TS: Tony Stone/ICL: Images Colour Library.

Photographer: Paul Postle
Hair & Make-up: Alison Butler
Make-up provided by: Screenface

Illustrations: Su Eaton

Fruit and vegetables: © 1996 PhotoDisc, Inc.
Author photograph: Chris Foster

INDEX